Visit www.springerpub.com to order.

FAST FACTS FOR THE FAITH COMMUNITY NURSE

Implementing FCN/Parish Nursing in a Nutshell

Janet S. Hickman, MS, EdD, RN, is a Professor of Nursing and has served as the interim Dean of Graduate Studies and Extended Education at West Chester University, West Chester, Pennsylvania, from 2006 to 2011. Dr. Hickman has a wide range of experience in nursing and nursing education spanning nearly 40 years. She has taught nursing at St. Joseph Hospital School of Nursing (Joliet, Illinois); Wright State University (Dayton, Ohio); Neuman College (Aston, Pennsylvania); and Eastern College (St. David's, Pennsylvania), and is currently teaching at West Chester University Department of Nursing (since 1992). Her MS is in Community Health Nursing, which she practiced as a VNA in Tarrytown, New York, and as Director of Home Care at Nyack (New York) Hospital. Her Doctor of Education degree is from Temple University (1986) in higher education administration. She has authored nursing journal articles and several textbook chapters, including texts published by W.B. Saunders and Prentice-Hall; and is the sole author of the textbook, *Faith Community Nursing*. She recently presented "Caring and Change" at the SE PA Chapter of Health Ministries Association. Dr. Hickman is a professional member of Sigma Theta Tau, Association of Community Health Nursing Educators, Council of Graduate Schools, Pennsylvania Council of Graduate Schools, North Atlantic Council of Graduate Schools, and National Association of Graduate Admissions Professionals.

FAST FACTS FOR THE FAITH COMMUNITY NURSE

Implementing FCN/Parish Nursing in a Nutshell

Janet S. Hickman, MS, EdD, RN

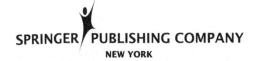
SPRINGER PUBLISHING COMPANY
NEW YORK

Springer Publishing Company, LLC
11 West 42nd Street
New York, NY 10036
www.springerpub.com

Acquisitions Editor: Margaret Zuccarini
Composition: Newgen Imaging

ISBN: **978-0-8261-0712-1**
eISBN: **978-0-8261-0713-8**

11 12 13 14 / 5 4 3 2 1

The author and the publisher of this Work have made every effort to use sources believed to be reliable to provide information that is accurate and compatible with the standards generally accepted at the time of publication. Because medical science is continually advancing, our knowledge base continues to expand. Therefore, as new information becomes available, changes in procedures become necessary. We recommend that the reader always consult current research and specific institutional policies before performing any clinical procedure. The author and publisher shall not be liable for any special, consequential, or exemplary damages resulting, in whole or in part, from the readers' use of, or reliance on, the information contained in this book. The publisher has no responsibility for the persistence or accuracy of URLs for external or third-party Internet Web sites referred to in this publication and does not guarantee that any content on such Web sites is, or will remain, accurate or appropriate.

Library of Congress Cataloging-in-Publication Data
Hickman, Janet Susan.
   Fast facts for the faith community nurse : implementing FCN/parish nursing
in a nutshell / Janet S. Hickman.
      p. ; cm.
   Includes bibliographical references and index.
   ISBN 978-0-8261-0712-1 — ISBN 978-0-8261-0713-8 (eISBN)
   1. Parish nursing. 2. Community health nursing. I. Title.
   [DNLM: 1. Spiritual Therapies—nursing. 2. Spirituality. 3. Community
Health Nursing—methods. 4. Holistic Nursing—methods. WY 87]
   RT120.P37H45 2011
   610.73'43—dc22   2011015447

Printed in the United States of America by Hamilton Printing.

Contents

Preface

This text was written for faith community nurses, from novices to experts. Special people are called to health ministry, and the goal of this book is to provide the information and resources necessary to be successful in the practice of faith community nursing. This specialty nursing practice combines the caring aspect of nursing with the spiritual and the sacred. It is an important and powerful combination in a time of decreased resources and health care system changes.

Part I provides an overview of faith community nursing practices—its roots, practice models, roles, and legal and ethical parameters. This is foundational information for all faith community nurses.

Part II includes chapters that inform the faith community nurse about initiating a faith community nursing ministry, assessing the health needs of the faith community, health education, teaching, and program planning and evaluation.

Part III presents information on meeting the special needs of the faith community and includes content on acute and chronic care needs, palliative care, and grief and loss. Additional chapters focus on connecting with community resources and vulnerable populations.

The format of this book is fast facts with extensive and clear paths to further information and helpful resource materials.

Janet S. Hickman, MS, EdD, RN

Acknowledgments

It is my pleasure to acknowledge the graduate nursing students at West Chester University who encouraged me to write about faith community nursing, as well as those nurses who practice in the field of faith community nursing. It is holistic nursing practice at its best!

I would like to acknowledge Margaret Zuccarini, Publisher, Nursing, Springer Publishing Company, as well as her editorial staff for their vision and technical excellence. Their support and assistance were essential to the success of this endeavor.

PART

Foundations

The Roots of Faith
Community Nursing

INTRODUCTION

Does the thought of working with a faith community appeal to you? Does the idea of working with people holistically, body and spirit, call to you in a way that a career in nursing does?

"Faith community nursing is the specialized practice of professional nursing that focuses on the intentional care of the spirit as part of the process of promoting holistic health and preventing or minimizing illness in a faith community" (American Nurses Association & Health Ministries Association [ANA–HMA], 2005, p. 1). A faith community nurse (FCN) is a licensed registered nurse who serves as a member of the faith community ministry staff. The FCN promotes health as wholeness to the members of the faith community in the context of the values, beliefs, and practices of the religious tradition. Faith community nursing is practiced in a wide variety of religious traditions in at least 15 countries.

In this chapter you will learn:

1. The practice of faith community nursing.
2. A brief history of faith community/parish nursing in the United States.
3. The philosophical basis for faith community nursing practice.
4. The importance of nursing theories in faith community nursing.

THE PRACTICE OF FAITH COMMUNITY NURSING

Faith community nursing is considered to be one of the newer specialties in nursing practice, yet the concepts underlying faith community nursing go back to the very roots of the nursing profession. Faith community nursing values the concepts of *caring, holism, health,* and *healing.* While *caring* has many definitions, it can be thought of as intentional attention to meeting the needs of another person. A *holistic* perspective views the person as a unified being with total integration of mind, body, and spirit. *Shalom*, God's intent for harmony and wholeness, serves as the foundation for understanding health (International Parish Nurse Resource Center [INPNRC], 2010). *Health* is "the integration of the physical, psychological, and social aspects of the patient to create a sense of harmony with self, others, the environment, and a higher power. Health may be experienced in the presence or absence of disease or injury" (ANA–HMA, 2005, pp. 2–3). *Healing* is "the process of integrating the mind, body, and spirit to bring about wholeness, health, and a sense of spiritual well-being, although the patient's disease may not be cured" (ANA–HMA, 2005, p. 3). In the language of this specialty, the patient is the recipient of nursing practice and may be an individual, family, or congregational community. *Congregational nurse* and *parish nurse* are earlier titles for this specialty, but all can be used interchangeably.

===*FAST FACTS in a NUTSHELL*

Elements for a Successful Faith
Community Nursing Program

• The support and endorsement—not just the permission—of the faith community leader and the ministry team.
• The ability of the structure to provide reliable long-term financial support for resources.
• The congregation's embracing of health and healing within its mission and organizational strategic planning. This includes program and personnel evaluation, and identifying and measuring program outcomes.
• The educational preparation of the FCN. The ANA–HMA recommends a bachelor of science in nursing (BSN) or higher degree, with academic preparation in community health nursing.

Educational expectations of the FCN differ from the IPNRC requirement of a registered nursing license and completion of the basic parish nurse course. This does not suggest that non-BSN-prepared parish nurses cannot be successful, but rather stresses the importance of preparation in community health nursing.

BRIEF HISTORICAL PERSPECTIVE

Nelson (1997) presents an excellent argument that "modern professional" nursing should be credited to the religious nursing sisters who practiced professional nursing before the Crimean War and the American Civil War. She states that the modern professional nurse cannot be seen as a product of secularization, but is an extension of a religious form of life. As Florence Nightingale viewed nursing as a spiritual enterprise within the context of a transcendent God, she would certainly agree with Nelson.

A professional strategy emphasizing efficiency, standard-ization, and scientific management characterized the devel-opment of nursing in the United States as early as the 19th century. The division of labor between care for the body and care for the soul, with care for the soul delegated to the clergy, became prevalent by the early 1920s.

The introduction of district nursing in the United States evolved into a distinctly American approach to home-based care characterized by both individualism and pluralism. Initially, public health nursing care was directed to sick, poor people in their homes and was funded by voluntary agencies such as visiting nurses associations, hospitals, and church groups. The mission emphasized health promotion and disease prevention rather than curative care. As local and state governments began to take responsibility for the health and welfare of their citi-zens, public health nursing services became part of local health departments. Delivery of services was directed to a wide spec-trum of people defined by geographic boundaries (e.g., cities and counties), special populations (e.g., maternal-child, adult health, and school health), and specific health problems, such as tuberculosis, venereal disease, and communicable diseases. As public secular structures replaced voluntary, church-related structures, the concept of holism in health care was lost.

In the first three decades of the 20th century, nursing-school graduates functioned as private duty nurses, instruc-tors, and public health nurses, as the care of the sick occurred in the home setting. American hospitals were staffed by stu-dent nurses who were supervised by a few graduate nurses. Their patients could not afford to be cared for at home (Baer, 1999). In the 1930s, the advances of science and technology moved the delivery of acute care from the home setting to the hospital. The need for nurses increased as hospitals grew and expanded their services. The delivery of nursing care became highly regimented and task-oriented, with attention to physical needs taking priority.

Barnum (2003) states that as nursing matured as an aspir-ing profession, it adopted the scientific paradigm. As a result, the focus of care moved from the holistic view of a person as a mind-body-spirit to that of a person as a biopsychosocial being. Nursing had to model itself after medicine and to accept the scientific paradigm to enter the turf of academia. Donley (1991) writes with concern about the loss of the art of nursing in response to technology and profit making: "As some of the art and most of the mystery of healing were lost, it became clear to nurses and others who worked in hospitals, that they were part of a technical money making system, not a sacred system" (p. 178). The focus of nursing had become curing, not caring.

During the 1950s and early 1960s, the "biopsychosocial era," nursing curricula were divested of spiritual content, which was replaced with content about the major world religions. Religious rituals and dietary practices were discussed in relation to nursing care, but the spiritual needs of the patient were referred to the appropriate clergy (Barnum, 2003).

Dr. Granger Westberg (1913–1999), a Lutheran minister, is considered the founder of parish nursing in the United States, or, as Kreutzer (2010) would argue, Westburg revived the practice of parish nursing. Westberg participated in a Kellogg Foundation–sponsored project that established medical clinics in Chicago churches staffed by physicians, nurses, and pastors in the 1970s. Evaluative data demonstrated that nursing could speak both the languages of science and religion. Westberg identified nursing as the "glue" that binds medicine and religion together for the patient. When funding for the clinics ended, Westberg suggested placing nurses in congregations as an alternative. Ultimately, the Lutheran General Hospital in Park Ridge, Illinois, subsidized the initial 6 pilot parish-nurse programs for a 3-year period (Westburg, 1999). Late in 1986, the IPNRC was established at the Lutheran General Health System (a predecessor of Advocate Health Care). Under the leadership of Ann Solari-Twadell, it became the lead organization for parish nurse education, research, and resource development. In 2001, Advocate Health Care closed the IPNRC and transferred its programs to Deaconess Parish Nurse Ministries in St. Louis, Missouri.

================================= *FAST FACTS in a NUTSHELL*

International Parish Nurse Resource Center

- Serves parish nurses worldwide and offers the annual Westberg Symposium as well as parish nurse preparation courses and resources for FCN practice.
- Provides a wealth of information on its website, (http://ipnrc.parishnurses.org/).
- Publishes a quarterly newsletter, *Parish Nurse Perspectives* (available by paid subscription) and periodic electronic IPNRC *eNotes*.

In 1989, the HMA was formed as an interfaith, multidisciplinary organization. The parish nurse section of HMA, in conjunction with the ANA, published the first edition of the *Scope and Standards of Parish Nursing Practice* in 1998. The second edition, entitled *Faith Community Nursing: Scope and Standards of Practice*, was published in 2005.

PHILOSOPHICAL BASIS FOR FAITH COMMUNITY NURSING PRACTICE

A philosophy is a set of beliefs about the nature, meaning, and important elements of something. A philosophy can be individual as well as organizational. The IPNRC's philosophy statement about parish nursing is presented in Figure 1.1.

Figure 1.1   IPNRC Philosophy of Parish Nursing

Parish nursing is a recognized specialty practice that combines professional nursing and health ministry. Parish nursing emphasizes health and healing within a faith community. The philosophy of

Continued

Figure 1.1 *Continued*

parish nursing embraces four major concepts: spiritual formation; professionalism; *shalom* as health and wholeness; and community, incorporating culture and diversity.

- **Spirit.** The spiritual dimension is central to parish nursing practice. Personal spiritual formation is an ongoing, essential component of practice for the parish nurse and includes both self-care and hospitality, through opening the heart to self and others. Spiritual formation is an intentional process of intimacy with God to foster spiritual growth.
- **Roots.** The parish nurse role reclaims the historic roots of professional nursing. Aspects of health and healing found in many faith traditions are embodied in the role of the parish nurse. The parish nurse practices under the scope and standards of practice and the ethical code of nursing as set forth in his or her country.
- *Shalom.* The parish nurse understands health to be a dynamic process that embodies the spiritual, psychological, physical, and social dimensions of the person. *Shalom*, God's intent for harmony and wholeness, serves as a foundation for understanding health. A sense of well-being can exist in the presence of imbalance, and healing can exist in the absence of cure.
- **Community.** The practice of parish nursing focuses on a faith community. The parish nurse, in collaboration with the pastoral staff and congregants, participates in the ongoing transformation of the

Continued

Figure 1.1   *Continued*

faith community into sources of health and healing. Through partnership with other community health resources, parish nursing fosters new and creative responses to health and wellness concerns. Parish nurses appreciate that all persons are sacred and must be treated with respect and dignity. The parish nurse serves the faith community, creates safe and sacred places for healing, and advocates with compassion, mercy, and dignity.

Source: http://www.parishnurses.org/Fundamentalsofpn.aspx#Philosophy of Parish Nursing

FAITH COMMUNITY NURSING AND NURSING THEORY

At its simplest, a theory provides direction in which to view facts and events. Polit and Beck (2008) define a theory as a systematic, abstract explanation of some aspect of reality. They state that in a theory, concepts are knitted together into a coherent system to describe or explain some aspect of the world. For example, Nightingale proposed a beneficial relationship between fresh air and health. Theories are based on assumptions that are presented as givens and must be viewed as "truths" because they cannot be empirically tested, as, for example, a value statement or an ethic. Theories can be presented as models in the form of a diagram or a map of the content (Hickman, 2011).

Why are nursing theories important to faith community nursing? The clear answer is that theories direct the acts and events that occur in nursing practice. In an applied discipline such as nursing, practice is based on theories that are validated by research, which in turn informs evidence-based practice.

Shelly and Miller (1999) strongly advocate for an explicitly Christian theology of nursing. They state that a Christian worldview cannot be superimposed on any other worldview. They define Christian nursing as "a ministry of compassionate care for the whole person, in response to God's grace toward a sinful world, which aims to foster optimum health (*shalom*) and bring comfort in suffering and death to anyone in need" (p. 18).

2

Looking at Holistic Health

INRODUCTION

The connections among faith, healing, wholeness, and faith communities are eternal. Every faith tradition explores the meaning of major life events.

In this chapter you will learn:

1. Concepts of holistic health.
2. Assumptions that underlie health and faith community nursing.
3. What research suggests about faith and health.

HEALTH

Traditional dictionary definitions of *health* present the idea of soundness in body, mind, and spirit, freedom from physical disease or pain, and well-being. Definitions of health are culturally bound and have evolved over time.

The Greek goddess Hygeia represented the idea that people could be healthy if they lived rationally. To the ancient Greeks, health was defined holistically and thought to be influenced by one's lifestyle and personal habits. Historically, physical wholeness and mental soundness were social expectations. Persons with disfiguring diseases, congenital anomalies, or inappropriate behaviors were ostracized from society because of the fear of contagion or that such persons harbored evil spirits (or both).

With the advent of germ theory, the causes of diseases were studied and understood in the terminology of science. Curing disease became a scientific and medical challenge. Because diseases were associated with specific microbial causes, being free of the causative agent defined health. Illness and health were viewed on a continuum as polar opposites. Physicians "ruled out" specific diseases to diagnose health.

The World Health Organization (WHO) Constitution (1948, p. 1) defines *health* as "a state of complete physical, mental, and social well-being and not merely the absence of disease and infirmity." The WHO definition of health has not been amended since 1948 and does not address spiritual health.

========*FAST FACTS in a NUTSHELL*

The WHO definition of *health* was revolutionary because it:

• Increased the number of components to consider in assessing health.
• Brought attention to the multidimensionality of health.
• Reflected concern for the individual as a total person.
• Placed health within the context of the social environment.
• Equated health with productive and creative living.

Source: Pender, Murdaugh, and Parson, 2002.

JUDEO-CHRISTIAN CONCEPTS OF HEALTH

Chase-Ziolek (2005) states that the Hebrew word *shalom* is considered the concept most related to the word *health* in the Bible. *Shalom* is often translated as "peace," but its meaning also encompasses prosperity, rest, safety, security, justice, happiness, and wholeness. Shelly and Miller (1999) concur, and add that *shalom* incorporates all the elements of a God-centered community. They state that a God-centered wholeness enables a person to live in harmony with self, God, and others, and to be responsible stewards of the environment.

Westberg (1982) made nine statements about health that he believed could be accepted by a wide variety of religious people. These statements appear in Figure 2.1.

Figure 2.1   Health According to Westberg (1982)

- Health is intimately related to how a person "thinketh in one's heart."
- Physical health is not our chief end in this life—only a possible by-product of loving God and one's neighbor as oneself.
- Health is closely tied up with goals, meaning, and purposeful living; it is a religious quest, whereas illness may be related to a life that is empty, bored, or without purpose or aim.
- Our present disease-oriented medical care system must be revised to include a strong accent on modeling and teaching prevention and wellness.
- Our present separation of body and spirit must go, and an integrated whole person approach must be put in its place.
- Merely existing is different than living under God and responding to the prompting of God's spirit.

Continued

> **Figure 2.1** *Continued*
>
> - The body functions at its best when a person, who is the body, exhibits attitudes of hope, love, and gratitude.
> - True health is closely associated with creativity by which we as people of God participate with God in the ongoing process of creation.
> - The self-preservation instincts of the human can happily be blended with the innate longing to love and to help others.

Westberg (1999) used the term *holistic health* to define a whole or completely integrated approach to health and health care that integrates the physical and spiritual aspects of the whole person. Jesus, in his ministry of healing, always dealt with people as whole persons. The principles of holistic health arose from the understanding that human beings strive for wholeness in relationship to God, themselves, their families, and society (American Nurses Association & Health Ministries Association [ANA–HMA], 2005). Nursing practice in the United States has come full circle, from a holistic approach to a biopsychosocial approach, and back to a holistic approach. When health is understood from an integrated perspective, the relationship between faith and health is apparent.

THE EASTERN PERSPECTIVE OF HEALTH

Eastern medical traditions are based on the premise that human beings are made up of energy systems and vital life force. The flow and balance of energy are the underlying principle of traditional Chinese medicine, Ayurvedic medicine, and other traditions. To maintain health, energy connecting the mind and body must be moving, flowing freely, and balanced. Lack of balance is believed to cause disease.

HEALTH AND FAITH COMMUNITY NURSING

The *Faith Community Nursing: Scope and Standards of Practice* (ANA–HMA, 2005) makes five assumptions that underlie faith community nursing:

- Health and illness are human experiences.
- Health is the integration of the spiritual, physical, psychological, and social aspects of the patient, promoting a sense of sense of harmony with self, others, the environment, and a higher power.
- Health may be experienced in the presence of disease or injury.
- The presence of illness does not preclude health, nor does optimal health preclude illness.
- Healing is the process of integrating the body, mind, and spirit to create wholeness, health, and a sense of well-being, even when the patient's illness is not cured. (pp. 3–4)

RESEARCH ABOUT FAITH AND HEALTH

In 1998, a landmark article appeared in the *Archives of Family Medicine* (Matthews, McCullough, Larson, Koenig, Swyers, & Milano) that reviewed the research literature about religious commitment and health status. The article reported that empirical data suggest that a religious commitment plays a beneficial role in preventing mental and physical illness, improving how people cope with illness, and facilitating recovery from illness. The authors suggest that health care practitioners who make several small changes in how patients' religious commitments are broached in clinical practice may enhance health outcomes.

Coyle (2002) suggests that people are better able to cope with or recover from illness when they feel they are not completely in control of their own destiny. Spirituality, based on transcendence or religious commitment, may provide the opportunity for a shared sense of responsibility through connectedness with a higher power.

3

Spiritual Caring

INRODUCTION

Through the use of spiritual histories and other tools, FCNs can understand the depth of patients' spiritual lives, which likely will affect their ability to cope with their health situations. Providing meaningful spiritual care involves one's own spiritual assessment, ministry of presence, observations of the patient's spirituality and ministry of the word.

In this chapter you will learn:

1. Concepts of spirituality.
2. Several different spiritual tools and assessments and how to use them,
3. Some guidelines for performing spiritual care.

SPIRITUALITY

Sessanna, Finnell, and Jezewski (2007) conducted a concept analysis of spirituality in nursing and health-related literature, reviewing 90 references. Concept analysis findings reveal that spirituality is defined within four main themes:

1. As religious systems of beliefs (spirituality equals religion)

2. As life meaning, purpose, and connection with others
3. As a nonreligious system of beliefs and values
4. As a metaphysical or transcendental phenomenon

Sessanna, Finnell, and Jezewski conclude that the definition of *spirituality* composed by Fowler and Peterson (1997) is the most inclusive, consistent with the findings resulting from their concept analysis. Figure 3.1 provides this definition.

From a Christian perspective, Dueck (2006) proposes the idea of thick and thin spirituality (Dueck & Reimer, 2003). In his view, thick spirituality is deep, contextual and nestled within a religious tradition and a faith community. This type of spirituality is a culturally rich, deep, and fully defined view of spiritual life. In contrast, he describes

Figure 3.1   Spirituality Defined by Fowler and
                Peterson (1997)

Spirituality is the way in which a person understands and lives life in view of her or his ultimate meaning, beliefs and values. It is the unifying and integrative aspect of the person's life and, when lived intentionally, is experienced as a process of growth and maturity. It integrates, unifies, and vivifies the whole of a person's narrative or story, embeds his or her core identity, establishes the fundamental basis for the individual's relationship with others and with society, includes a sense of the transcendent, and is the interpretative lens through which the person sees the world. It is the basis for community for it is in spirituality that we experience our co-participation in the shared human condition. It may or may not be expressed in religious categories (p. 47).

nonreligious spirituality as "thin" and shallow, and not rooted in any tradition.

═══════════════════════════*FAST FACTS in a NUTSHELL*

Dueck's Criticisms of Thin Spirituality

• **It is utilitarian.** This is a problem because it is used simply because it works and can be used by anyone. To value spirituality for its usefulness is a form of idolatry (p. 5).
• **It is consumerist.** It views spirituality as a commodity, with the risk that it can be bought and sold.
• **It is private and within the individual, devoid of community.**

SPIRITUAL HISTORIES

Since 2000, the Joint Commission (JC) has mandated that all clients be assessed for spiritual beliefs and practices and have available spiritual support. Over the years, several spiritual assessment and history tools have been developed by nurses, physicians, and chaplains. While the language of the various disciplines differs, it is generally accepted that a **spiritual screen** is performed at most institutions upon admission of the patient. According to LaRocca-Pitts (2008), a screen consists of one or two questions aimed at determining a person's particular religion or faith and whether there are any specific spiritual, religious or cultural needs the hospital can address. A **spiritual history**, on the other hand, seeks to understand how a person's spiritual life might affect his or her ability to cope with the health situation he or she is facing. A spiritual history is brief, and generally includes no more than four or five questions. The information gained via the history is subject to change as diagnosis, prognosis, and treatment plans evolve. If a spiritual history presents concerns, an in-depth spiritual assessment is recommended.

Koenig recommends that spiritual history tools be brief, memorable, appropriate, patient-centered, and credible.

==*FAST FACTS in a NUTSHELL*

Three of the more commonly used spiritual history tools:

1. **Koenig's (2002) spiritual history tool** uses the acronym CSI-MEMO.

   CS – Do your religious/spiritual beliefs provide Comfort, or are they a source of Stress?

   I – Do you have spiritual beliefs that might Influence your medical decision?

   MEM – Are you a MEMber of a religious or spiritual community, and is it supportive to you?

   O – Do you have any Other spiritual needs you'd like someone to address?

2. **Puchalski and Romer's (2000) spiritual history tool** uses the acronym FICA.

   F – Faith, Belief, Meaning.

   I – Importance or Influence of religious and spiritual beliefs and practices.

   C – Community or Church connections.

   A – Address/Action in the context of medical care.

3. **Larocca-Pitts (2008) spiritual history tool** uses the acronym FACT.

   F – Faith or Beliefs: What is your Faith or belief? Do you consider yourself a person of Faith or a spiritual person? What things do you believe give your life meaning and purpose?

   A – Active (or Available, Accessible, Applicable): Are you Active in your faith community? Is support for your faith Available to you? Do you have Access to what you need to Apply your faith?

   C – Coping, Conflicts or Concerns: How are you coping with your medical situation? Is your faith helping you to cope? How is your faith

Continued

Continued

> providing comfort? Are any of your beliefs in
> Conflict with medical treatment? Do you have
> Concerns?
>
> T – Treatment Plan: Based on the responses to these
> questions, the clinician makes a judgment as to
> the appropriate Treatment plan.

SPIRITUAL ASSESSMENT

Spiritual assessment tools developed by nurses include:

- *The Spiritual Perspective Scale*, which measures adult spiritual views (Reed, 1991).
- *The Spiritual Assessment Tool*, developed to identify the spiritual needs of nursing-home residents (Kerrigan & Harkulich, 1993).
- *The Spiritual Well-Being Scale*, a tool to assess the spiritual attitudes of older adults (Hungelmann, Kenkel-Rossi, Klassen, & Stollenwerk, 1996).
- *The Spiritual Needs Survey*, which includes seven major constructs: belonging, meaning, hope, the sacred, morality, beauty, and acceptance of dying (Galek, Flannelly, Vane, & Galek, 2005).
- *The Spiritual Assessment Model*, with five constructs (Dameron, 2005).
- *The Spiritual Assessment Scale (SAS)* contains 21 items of 3 subscales: Personal Faith, Religious Practice, and Spiritual Contentment (O'Brien, 2008).

SPIRITUAL CARE

Carson and Koenig (2004) developed guidelines for providing spiritual care:

- *Spiritual self–assessment:* Are you spiritually aware? Do you spend time with God in reflection, in prayer?

- *Ministry of presence:* Listen carefully to hear the person's story and look for patterns. Provide a ministry of presence, which requires empathy, vulnerability, humility, and commitment.
- *Observe:*
  - *Nonverbal behavior:* What emotion(s) does it convey?
  - *Verbal behavior:* References made to God, prayer, faith, hope, religion.
  - *Interpersonal relationships:* Does the person have supportive family and friends?
  - *The environment:* Are religious items apparent?
- *Ministry of the Word:*
  - A willingness to discuss spiritual/religious issues.
  - Verbal support and encouragement of spiritual beliefs (e.g., making a referral to a chaplain, using scripture or other religious literature, using prayer).
- *Ministry of Action:* How you do what you do? The simplest acts can convey caring and love.

THE ROLE OF PRESENCE IN SPIRITUAL CARE

The nursing intervention of presence is defined by the Nursing Intervention Classification (NIC) as "being with another, both physically and psychologically, during times of need" (Cavendish et al., 2003, p. 120).

═══════════════════════*FAST FACTS in a NUTSHELL*

Nursing activities in the intervention of presence include:

- Demonstrating an accepting attitude.
- Verbally communicating empathy.
- Establishing trust and a positive regard.
- Listening to the patient's concerns.

Continued

Continued
- Touching the patient to express concern as appropriate.
- Being physically available as a helper.
- Remaining physically present without expecting interactional responses.

In her nursing theory of human becoming, Parse (1998, 2007) describes "true presence" as the way nurses interact with patients with the goal of improving quality of life. True presence can be implemented by fact-to-face dialogue, by silent immersion, and by lingering presence (involving memories and reflection). A nurse practicing true presence is nonjudgmental and takes all cues from the patient. When the nurse is truly present with the patient, the patient defines health. The concept of true presence is valuable to faith community nursing practice. Hearing the voice of the patient without imposing one's own values is paramount.

NURSING RESEARCH

Van Dover and Pfeiffer (2006) conducted a qualitative research study to explore and describe the processes that Christian parish nurses used as they gave spiritual care. From its initial emergence as the core category, "Bringing God Near" became a Basic Social Process theory of giving spiritual care for the parish nurses. Sequential phases within the process include trusting God, forming a relationship with the patient and family, opening up to God, activating and nurturing faith, and recognizing spiritual renewal.

Deal's (2008) research on the lived experience of giving spiritual care supports Van Dover and Pfeiffer's findings. While the study subjects were dialysis nurses, not parish nurses, similar themes emerged. Deal identified five themes: "Drawing close," "Drawing from the well of my spiritual resources," "The pain of spiritual distress," "Lack of resources to give spiritual care," and "Giving spiritual care is like diving down deep." These findings illuminated nurses' experiences of giving spiritual care as a continuum dependent upon the needs of the patient, and suggest that nurses and patients draw close during the giving of spiritual care and also that giving spiritual care can have an emotional cost.

4

Faith Community Nursing Models of Delivery

INTRODUCTION

Different structures meet the needs of faith communities and the larger communities in which they reside. In addition to several models of the practice of faith community nursing, there are four models through which faith community nursing practice is delivered: the institutional model, the congregational paid model, the congregational volunteer model, and the paid consortium model.

In this chapter you will learn:

1. Several models of faith community nursing practice.
2. The four models of delivery of faith community nursing delivery.

MODELS OF FAITH COMMUNITY NURSING PRACTICE

Berquist and King (1994) presented the first conceptual model of parish nursing. They describe the patient as a physiological, emotional, and spiritual person. Health is defined as optimal wellness and wholeness. The faith community is the environment in which the parish nurse practices. Parish nursing practice includes the roles of health educator, health counselor, leader of groups, and community liaison. The goal of parish nursing in this model is to enhance the holistic health and well-being of the faith community members.

Bunkers (1998, 1999) and Putnam (1995) describe a nursing theory-guided model of health ministry and parish nursing practice at the First Presbyterian Church in Sioux Falls, South Dakota, that is based on Parse's theory of human becoming in parallel with the Beatitudes. The model was created because it focuses on quality of life from the person's/parish's perspective, and it uses the strengths and resources within the church as a foundation for providing care. A parish nurse practicing within this theory is open to how others choose to live, without judging their choices.

The Miller Model (1997) for Parish Nursing is based on the theological perspective of evangelical Christianity and contains four elements: person/parishioner, health, parish nurse, and community/parish. The core integrating concept of the Miller Model is the Triune God. Health and healing are integral to a Christian church's mission and ministry.

=====*FAST FACTS in a NUTSHELL*

The Miller Model for Parish Nursing as Diagrammed in Three Stained-Glass Windows

1. The components and major concepts of the model: The Triune God surrounded by health, parish nurse, community and parishioner, ministry, dependence, mission, confession, communion, dignity, *shalom-*wholeness, and stewardship.
2. The aspects of a whole person and health-promoting resources.
3. The contexts of the parish nurse's role.

Wilson (1997) created the Parish Nurse Continuity of Care Model, which emphasizes harmony in mind, body, and spirit. It depicts "the nurse as the focal point of the model who connects individuals and families with resources to provide care to a congregation over life's continuum: physical birth, new life—being born again in Christ, suffering—the pains and sorrows of life, surrender—to God's grace and mercy, physical death and resurrection—everlasting life in glory with Christ" (p. 94).

Maddox (2001) provides a model called the Circle of Christian Caring, in which parish nursing is envisioned as "an opportunity to combine the spiritual and physical dimensions of caregiving and to affirm the church as a place for disease prevention and health promotion" (p. 12). Parish nurse roles are health educator, health counselor, referral/resource/client advocate, facilitator/leader, and home visitor.

Davis Lee (2006) developed a personal theory of Christian nursing based on her experiences as a nurse. She examined three poignant cases from her practice and used an inductive process to develop concepts to advance her own understanding of her nursing practice. The major concepts in Davis Lee's theory are based on Jesus' exemplary life. The caring relationship between the nurse and patient flow from the nurse's relationship with Jesus. The theory shows how world stressors such as illness and suffering can create feelings of futility, hopelessness, and helplessness, which lead to a cry for help. Jesus exemplifies the Christian attributes of connection, communication, caring solace, watchful knowing, honesty, facing fear, waiting, acknowledging grief, and duty, all of which a Christian nurse can use to provide care.

MODELS OF FAITH COMMUNITY NURSING DELIVERY

There are four major models of faith community or parish nursing: the Institutional Model, the Paid Congregational

Model, the Unpaid or Volunteer Congregational Model, and the Paid Consortium Model.

Institutional Model

The original parish-nurse pilot project, coordinated by Rev. Granger Westburg with Lutheran General Hospital, was an institutional model in which the hospital employed parish nurses. The congregations shared part of the cost of service based on a contractual agreement between the churches and the hospital (1990).

Many parish nursing programs were established in the 1990s, when hospitals and health care systems were seeking community-based partnerships. This was a time of intense competition for clients and provided a marketing tool for health care providers. The institutional model can be entirely owned and operated by a health care provider system, or the provider can employ coordinators who help individual congregations set up parish nursing programs, using paid or unpaid nurses, and provide resources and consultation to church-based parish nurses.

The institutional model is most often hospital- or health-system directed; however, long-term care facilities and community agencies also have faith community nursing programs. When an institutional model is driven solely by economics as opposed to mission, economic downturns lead to the discontinuation of such programs. When the programs mesh with the mission of the health care provider, they are seen as cost-effective services to vulnerable populations.

In the institutional model, an FCN is a paid employee of the health care provider and may or may not be a member of the faith community served. The mission, goals, and outcomes are determined by the employing institution and thus take priority over those of the faith community. For some faith communities, incompatible missions between the health care provider and congregation are unacceptable.

An obvious advantage of the institutional model is the depth of the institution's resources. For the FCN, this means paid employment with benefits, institutional liability coverage, a network of peers across the system, professional development opportunities, and travel reimbursement. For the program, it means availability of health supplies and literature, referral opportunities, uniform documentation of client services, and access to interdisciplinary consultation.

Smith (2000, 2003) calls the institutional model the "marketplace model" and argues that the term *parish nurse* is inappropriate in this model because secular nurses deliver programs planned by their employers rather than the congregation, and that the church setting is merely the venue. She believes that secular nurses in churches are not the same as Christian nurses doing ministry as insider-experts in their own congregations.

Schumann's (2000) response to Smith's argument is that there are many secular institutions that advocate for holistic health, including spiritual health. In promoting spiritual wellness, institutions do contribute to the overall well-being of the community by helping churches to care for the Christian family in a Godly way. This is an ecumenical view that allows for a diversity of faith traditions to benefit from faith community nursing. There are merits to both points of view.

Paid Congregational Model

In the paid congregational model of faith community nursing, the FCN is a paid member of the ministry team and is accountable to the congregational leader, as well as to a board or council. The FCN has a spiritual call to serve in a ministry role, and authority for the position comes from being called by God to the ministry and by being endorsed or installed by the congregation. Solari-Twadell and Hackbarth (2010) report that 31% of parish nurses serve in paid positions.

Smith (2000, 2003) believes that the congregational model (paid or unpaid) is the only model deserving the title *faith community nurse,* as its Christian ministry aspect of faith community nursing is paramount.

Patterson (2003) describes the paid congregational model as ministry in the manner of Peter. The apostles in the early Christian church were told to take no money, but to accept provisions from those to whom they ministered. This is one of the tenets underlying the practice of providing salaries for ordained clergy.

═══════════════════════════════FAST FACTS in a NUTSHELL

Patterson's (2003) Factors Favoring a Paid Parish Nurse Program Within a Congregation

- **Professional health ministry:** Paying parish nurses underscores the message that parish nursing is a professional ministry of the church, requiring professional education and expertise.
- **Expectations and supervision:** A paid FCN is supervised as an employee and held to a standard job description as a term of employment.
- **Increased time commitment:** A paid FCN may have fewer distractions and will not be forced to seek full-time employment elsewhere.
- **Confidentiality:** A paid FCN is perceived as a professional on the ministry team, rather than a member of the congregation "wearing two hats."
- **Larger pool of applicants:** Compensation increases the chances of having a pool of applicants from which to choose.
- **Increased visibility:** Inclusion of a faith community nursing program in the congregational budget ensures wide support of such a ministry.

Unpaid or Volunteer Congregational Model

While the literature endorses the paid model of faith community nursing practice as the ideal, Solari-Twadell and Hackbarth (2010) report that 68% of practicing parish nurses are unpaid. **In the unpaid or volunteer congregational model, the FCN is considered part of the congregation's ministry team but serves without compensation.** The FCN's job description and selection are determined by the congregation's organizational structure.

The part-time volunteer model of faith community nursing is most common. Part-time and retired nurses function effectively as voluntary FCNs while maintaining all aspects of professional nursing standards. Many FCNs see advantages and flexibility in this model.

═══════════════════════════*FAST FACTS in a NUTSHELL*

Smith's (2003) Areas of Concern Related to the Volunteer Model

1. **Church volunteers have lower status than ministry staff.** The term *ministry staff* denotes mutual expectations of both the church and the nurse, whereas responsibilities are negotiable when the term *volunteer* is used.
2. **Pastoral and administrative support are decreased.** The pastoral leadership must give visible support for the faith community nursing program and clearly tie it to the missions of the congregation.
3. **There is inadequate professional accountability.** While a volunteer FCN has a call to serve, this does not negate professional responsibilities to public regulations and nursing practices.

Patterson (2003) describes unpaid or volunteer parish nursing as a ministry in the manner of the apostle Paul, who maintained his tent-making work to support himself financially in his outreach ministry. While Patterson endorses the paid model as optimal, she does present factors that can argue for an unpaid program within a congregation.

==========FAST FACTS in a NUTSHELL

*Patterson's (2003) Factors Favoring an
Unpaid Program Within a Congregation*

- **A priesthood of all believers:** All members of the church are called to be ministers, and the unpaid parish nurse affirms this.
- **Installation and recognition:** These apply to unpaid and paid nurses.
- **Ease of program start-up:** It is easier to start a program with a volunteer than to add a line item to the church budget.
- **Established presence in the church:** As a church member, a volunteer FCN may have a head start on the congregation's needs and concerns.
- **Lower cost to the congregation.**

Patterson also points out that it is difficult to terminate volunteers and suggests that they have clear job descriptions. Volunteers also may feel free to take extended vacations at any time, so the coverage issue should be addressed at the outset.

Paid Consortium Model

In the paid consortium model of faith community nursing, **the FCN is paid by a consortium of faith communities.** The FCN may divide her or his time equally among the congregations in the consortium, or the FCN may develop a health program that rotates the delivery setting among congregations to share resources.

New Models

Because of the economic constraints of today's world, faith communities and health care providers will creatively design new models of delivering faith-based nursing care. In addition to the various collaborative partnerships between churches and health care systems, university schools and colleges of nursing seek faith community nursing clinical placement for students. These collaborative partnerships extend and expand services to congregations as well as meet the learning needs of nursing students (Otterness, Gehrke, & Sener, 2007).

5

Exploring Faith Community Nursing Roles

INTRODUCTION

Faith community nurses take on a variety of roles in their practice. The original seven parish nurse roles were identified and described by Dr. Westburg. Recent nursing research identifies different FCN roles, all of which are related to spiritual care.

In this chapter you will learn:

1. Preparation for faith community nursing and the standards of practice.
2. The original seven parish nurse roles.
3. FCN roles supported by recent research about faith community nursing practice.

WHAT MAKES A FCN?

Faith Community Nursing: Scope and Standards of Practice (ANA–HMA, 2005) discusses the preferred minimum preparation for the specialty practice of faith community nursing. This preparation should include:

- A BSN or higher nursing degree and academic preparation in community nursing.
- Experience as a registered nurse (RN) using the nursing process.
- Knowledge of the health care assets of the community.
- Detailed knowledge of the spiritual beliefs and practices of the faith community.
- Specialized knowledge and skills to practice faith community nursing.

Standards of Practice

In 1986, the International Parish Nurse Resource Center (IPNRC) was founded to guide the parish nurse movement and to standardize the practice of parish nursing. In 1987, the IPNRC offered its first parish nursing education courses. It is estimated that over 12,000 nurses have completed this standardized core curriculum, called the basic preparation course (IPNRC, 2010). As completion of this curriculum is voluntary and may not be required by congregations, it is not possible to know how many practicing parish nurses there actually are. The IPNRC Website provides assumptions for parish nurse practice and curricula. These include:

- The participant is an RN with a current license or a student in a BSN program.
- The practice is considered a calling in which ministry shapes the practice.
- The practice encourages a partnership between parish nurses and individuals, families, faith communities, and the larger communities across the life span.
- The practice values the professional standards of the country in which it occurs.
- The curriculum focuses on core concepts of spirituality, professionalism, *shalom,* as health and wholeness, and community, incorporating culture and diversity.

- The curriculum is developed from a Judeo-Christian theological framework of care and is applicable to and respectful of other faith traditions.
- The curriculum develops nurses for leadership roles in collaborative health ministry.
- The curriculum supplies the content to develop and sustain parish nursing practice and individual spiritual growth (www.parishnurses.org/, 2010).

The IPNRC partners with educational providers around the country to offer a baccalaureate level, 36-hour, basic preparation course that provides core parish nurse content. The course may be offered for college credit or as continuing education.

═══════════════════════════════════*FAST FACTS in a NUTSHELL*

Content of the IPNRC Basic Preparation Course

- History and philosophy of parish nursing.
- Prayer, self-care, and healing and wholeness.
- Ethical issues, documenting practice, and legal aspects.
- Beginning one's ministry.
- Communication and collaboration, health promotion, and transforming life issues.
- Community assessment and accessing resources.
- Advocacy and care coordination.

The IPNRC also offers coordinator-preparation and faculty-preparation courses, and continuing education modules for parish nurses. The IPNRC Website provides a list of educational partners, locations, and schedules for course offerings. A coordinator's manual is available for a fee. The IPNRC courses value process dynamics in the educational process to allow for deep personal engagement of the learners and to provide opportunities to develop networks with others. Hospitality is a process dynamic for the creation of a safe, sacred space where others are welcomed. The character of the space, the religious nature, and the reflective demeanor of the learners draw attention to spirituality, the core of faith community nursing practice.

Professional Performance Standard 8: Education of *Faith Community Nursing: Scope and Standards of Practice* recommends that FCNs attain knowledge and competency that reflect current nursing practice.

══════════════════════════*FAST FACTS in a NUTSHELL*

Criteria for FCN Professional Performance Standard 8: Education

- Participates in ongoing educational activities related to spiritual care, professional nursing practice, and related professional issues.
- Demonstrates commitment to lifelong learning thorough self-reflection and inquiry to identify learning needs.
- Seeks learning experiences that reflect current practice to maintain and acquire knowledge, skills, and competence in all dimensions of faith community nursing.
- Maintains professional records providing evidence of competency in the specialty.
- Uses current research findings and other evidence to expand knowledge and enhance role performance to provide spiritual care.

The American Nurses Credentialing Center (ANCC) recently announced some new expectations for the certification/recognition of any nursing specialty. These expectations involve a minimum association size and the financial resources necessary for ongoing involvement with the ANCC. Both the HMA and IPNRC are committed to working jointly to meet ANCC expectations.

FCN ROLES

Westburg (1990, 1999) identified seven nonprioritized roles for the parish nurse: integrator of faith and health, personal health counselor, health educator, health advocate, referral agent, coordinator of volunteers, and developer of support groups. The roles that the FCN assumes in the work setting are dependent upon many factors. Clearly, time is a factor that can limit the number of roles any FCN can actualize. The needs of the congregation, the presence or absence of a health ministry team, and the personal preferences and priorities of the FCN will all affect how the roles are prioritized.

Integrator of Faith and Health

The integrator of faith and health role of the FCN is the overarching role of faith community nursing practice. It is faith community nursing in a nutshell. Every contact made by the FCN assists a person to strengthen his or her spiritual life to become and stay more whole and healthy. To actualize this role, the FCN needs to be knowledgeable about the human spirit, spirituality, and how spirituality and religion overlap, in the context of the faith tradition of the congregation. Practice in this role requires both spiritual maturity and openness to spiritual growth on the part of the FCN. Spiritual assessment skills are required, and spiritual resources need to be in place for referrals. Spiritual interventions are developed collaboratively with other members of the congregation's ministry team. Spiritual resources may include prayer, music, worship, sacraments, and healing rituals (Hickman, 2006).

Dahl (2010) states that an FCN aids in the transformation of the faith community into a source of health by building on people's strengths and guiding them in caring for themselves and for each other. Caiger (2006) suggests that this is accomplished through the process of *walking alongside* the person in need of care, which is the provision of support to the person while not taking over.

FAST FACTS in a NUTSHELL

Those who seek faith community nursing services:

* Are often in some form of crisis or life transition.
* Need introspection as well as reflection to understand and cope with their situation.
* May question their faith and/or voice doubt.
* With active listening by and presence of the FCN, can be helped to use the situation to further grow in their faith, and thus in overall health.

For congregants who are not experiencing any form of crisis, the FCN may act as a role model for them to open themselves more fully to incorporate holiness into their lives through reflection and prayer.

Personal Health Counselor

FCNs spend much of their time in the personal health counselor role. As such, FCNs assess the health needs of individuals, families, and the congregation, and provide appropriate interventions. Personal health counseling is related to health promotion and disease prevention.

Personal health counseling can occur as a planned activity, but it very often happens informally during health screening events, home visits, hospital visits, and nursing home visits. Personal counseling helps people express their feelings, identify health issues of concern and possible ways to deal with them, and evaluates the effectiveness of newly learned skills and behaviors.

Health Educator

Acting in the health educator role, FCNs provide the faith community with opportunities to participate in well-organized seminars, workshops, health fairs, classes and discussion groups covering a wide range of wellness and health topics. Health education is an appropriate activity for the faith community as people view their health through the lens of their faith tradition. Many people view wellness and health as good stewardship.

Often, a congregational assessment will direct the FCN in types of health education to offer. The FCN may provide educational programming or coordinate it with experts from the congregation or the larger community. Assessment data also direct the days and times that are convenient for the target audiences. Health education programming can also serve as a means for case finding for FCNs. These events may set the stage for follow-up home visits or phone contacts.

Knowledge of the principles of teaching and learning assists FCNs to be successful in health education. Attention should be paid to literacy levels of materials provided to participants as well as to age appropriateness. All programs should include measurable learning outcomes that can later be used in the evaluation process.

===*FAST FACTS in a NUTSHELL*

The Health Educator Role

- Spans a spectrum from one-on-one teaching to providing a congregational program.
- Includes making sure that information provided is current and accurate.
- Includes sermons, children's story times, and health fairs to provide health education.
- Shares information through bulletin boards, pamphlets, and poster displays, in newsletters, bulletin inserts, and on the congregational Web page.

Health Advocate

Patterson (2007) identifies eight advocacy roles for the FCN:

1. *Help parishioners obtain access to care* by connecting them with health insurance and public assistance.

2. *Serve as a health navigator* by helping parishioners understand what questions to ask to be fully informed about their options for services and treatment.
3. *Serve as a patient advocate in the health care system* by monitoring patient care and encouraging patients and families to speak up about their concerns.
4. *Work to acquire needed services in a community.*
5. *Mobilize for health of neighbors,* such as offering life skills and/or parenting classes.
6. *Raise awareness of legislative issues related to health* by encouraging political action.
7. *Advocate for environmental concerns* such as lead-poisoning prevention.
8. *Work for others in developing countries.*

Advocacy is part of each of the FCN roles and is based on the belief that all persons are sacred and should be treated with respect and dignity. In the advocate role, FCNs work with individuals, the faith community, and all available resources to provide whatever is in the best interests of holistic health. Reinhard, Grossman, and Piren (2004) state that nurses' ethical responsibility is to transfer as much knowledge as possible to patients and to support them in making informed choices. Advocacy can be teaching, nonjudgmental support of a person's decisions, and assistance in acting on those choices. FCNs listen and learn the needs of patients, assist them in making informed decisions, and speak for them when they are unable to do so themselves. The advocacy role is well supported by research findings related to faith community nursing roles and is clearly articulated in *Faith Community Nursing: Scope and Standards of Practice.*

Referral Agent

In the referral agent role, FCNs provide and document referrals to health care and social services available within the faith community and in the external community. In this role, FCNs match the needs of congregants with appropriate and available resources. Follow-up with congregants about the effectiveness of and satisfaction with services used is important as well.

Developer of Support Groups

Faith communities share beliefs and values, and their members come together to worship and support each other in those beliefs. FCNs may formalize support groups to meet various needs within the congregation. Examples include a caregiver group, a weight-management group, and a grief and loss group. Hurley and Mohnkern (2004) describe this role more fully.

Coordinator of Volunteers

In the coordinator of volunteers role, FCNs train and coordinate laypersons to extend the helping ministries of the faith community. Olson (2000) believes that facilitating volunteer activities is one way to ensure that the health ministry belongs to the greater congregation. Examples of volunteer health ministry activities include transportation services, foster grandparents, friendly visitor programs, and outreach programs. The FCN collaborates with congregational volunteers, assesses needs, and serves as a clinical resource.

Sage (2008) describes a resource notebook for volunteers that includes names and addresses of homebound members, visit records, laminated scripture cards, guidelines for hospital visits, and an inventory of medical equipment that could be loaned out. Sage stresses that volunteers must be well matched with care receivers and have the necessary training and support. A new resource available for FCNs is *The Volunteer Book: A Guide for Churches and Non-Profits.*

Current research findings do not identify the role of coordinator of volunteers as being central to faith community nursing practice. As the majority of FCNs serve in unpaid positions, the function of this role has lower priority than others.

SCOPE AND STANDARDS OF PRACTICE

Faith Community Nursing: Scope and Standards of Practice (ANA–HMA, 2005, pp. x–xi) defines roles of the FCN in a nursing process format:

1. **Assessment**: The FCN collects comprehensive data pertinent to the patient's holistic health or the situation.
2. **Diagnosis**: The FCN analyzes the holistic assessment data to determine the diagnoses or issues.
3. **Outcomes Identification**: The FCN identifies expected outcomes for a plan individualized to the patient or the situation.
4. **Planning**: The FCN develops a plan that prescribes strategies and alternatives to attain expected outcomes for individuals, families or the faith community as a whole.
5. **Implementation**: The FCN implements the plan by:
   a. Coordinating care
   b. Providing health teaching and/or health promotion
   c. Consulting
6. **Evaluation**: The FCN evaluates progress to outcome attainment.
7. **Collaboration**: The FCN collaborates with the patient, spiritual leaders, members of the faith community, and others in the conduct of practice.

New Definitions of FCN Roles

Solari-Twadell and Hackbarth (2010) conducted the largest study to date of parish nurses. The purposes of this study were to:

- Generate a comprehensive national data set describing parish nursing in the United States to provide an evidence base for a new paradigm of the ministry of parish nursing practice.
- Use data provided by parish nurses as objective evidence to establish what parish nurses are actually doing to promote the health of their faith communities.

- Assess what parish nurses believe is the "essence" or core of their practice.

The study had a demographic section (the findings of which were presented in Chapter 1). A second component consisted of the survey based on the Nursing Intervention Classification (NIC) developed by the Iowa Intervention Project Research Team (1996). The NIC survey tool contained 486 nursing interventions representing seven domains and 30 classes (McCloskey & Bulechek, 2000). An additional section allowed respondents to indicate which interventions they believed to be essential or core to the specialty practice. The final tool had 602 items and took approximately 2.5 hours to complete.

Solari-Twadell and Hackbarth used the list of 4,000 parish nurses who had completed the basic training course between 1997 and 2000. Every one of these nurses who had an accurate address and was currently practicing as a parish nurse was invited to participate (*n* = 2330). There were 1,161 useable surveys returned, for a response rate of 54%.

Study Findings

The majority of frequently used interventions belonged in five domains:

1. *Behavioral Domain:* "Care that supports psychosocial functioning and facilitates lifestyle changes" including:
   - Active listening.
   - Presence, touch, spiritual support, emotional support, spiritual growth facilitation, hope instillation, humor, and counseling.
   - Religious ritual enhancement, truth telling, values clarification, assisting others to gain self-awareness, and support in decision making.
2. *Health System Domain:* "Care that supports effective use of the health care delivery system" including:
   - Documentation

- Telephone consultation
- Telephone follow-up
3. *Family Domain:* "Care that supports the family unit" including:
   - Caregiver support
4. *Safety Domain:* "Care that supports protection form harm" including:
   - Health screening
   - Vital-signs monitoring
5. *Community Domain:* "Care that supports the health of the community" including:
   - Program development

Solari-Twadell and Hackbarth summarize these findings by stating that "Unique to the practice of parish nursing is the frequent use of the interventions of presence, touch, spiritual support, spiritual growth facilitation, and hope instillation. In addition, the more common nursing interventions of active listening, emotional support, and health education are prominent" (p. 72). They further find Westburg's seven functions of parish nursing to be limiting, and recommend that these no longer be used as a primary description of the ministry of parish nursing practice. Data from their study suggest a new definition of the ministry of parish nursing practice as care that supports and facilitates:

- Physical functioning
- Psychological functioning and lifestyle changes, with particular emphasis on coping assistance and spiritual care
- Protection against harm; the family unit; effective use of the health care system; and health of the congregation and community (p. 74)

Solari-Twadell and Hackbarth suggest that their findings be used to inform future revisions of the professional Scope and Standards document for faith community nursing, as well as curricular revisions in parish nurse preparation.

6

Practicing Faith Community Nursing Within Legal Parameters

INTRODUCTION

There are legal aspects of faith community nursing practice. While there have been no successful lawsuits against FCNs, they are held to the same standards of practice as are all RNs. Elements of those standards include accountability, nurse practice acts, confidentiality, and documentation.

In this chapter you will learn:

1. Legal accountability and liability in faith community nursing.
2. Documentation and other legal parameters of faith community nursing.

ACCOUNTABLILITY

To be accountable is to answer for one's professional judgment and actions within a frame of authority. In the faith community setting, the FCN's job description addresses accountability by clearly describing the duties, responsibilities, and expectations of the position. The job description should clearly state to whom the FCN is accountable and the expected frequency and specificity of reporting. Several formal documents address the accountability of FCNs. State nurse practice acts (NPAs) mandate educational requirements for RN licensure and the legal scope of practice of professional nurses. All FCNs must hold an active RN license in the state in which they practice, and this requirement should be included in all FCN job descriptions. All nurses should be familiar with the NPA in their state, as well as accompanying rules and regulations. Exceeding the scope of practice defined in NPAs invites legal action against the practitioner. All state boards of nursing maintain Websites where changes to NPAs are posted.

Standards of care set expected criteria for job proficiency so that both nurses and others can judge the quality of care provided. Although standards of care are guidelines, not laws, they are used in courts to provide expectations for practice. Authority for the practice of nursing is based on a social contract recognizing the professional rights and responsibilities of nursing and of public accountability. *Nursing's Social Policy Statement* (American Nurses Association [ANA], 2010b) discusses the profession's relationship with society and its obligation to patients. FCNs also practice according to *Faith Community Nursing: Scope and Standards of Practice* (American Nurses Assocation & Health Ministries Assocation [ANA–HMA], 2005), which sets higher standards than minimum nursing credentials.

Van Loon and Carey (2002) note the mutual accountability that parish nurses have with members of the ministerial team "for work being clearly defined, fairly delegated and appropriately shared (p. 151). O'Brien (2003) discusses the importance of documentation to protect the faith community, provide evidence of the usefulness of the program, and document its outcomes on the lives of faith community members. Smith (2003) suggests that FCNs increase their program accountability by developing appropriate written policies, including policies defining who is eligible for the services of the FCN, documentation, confidentiality, scope of practice, medical emergencies in the home, death in the home, safety of FCNs, and infectious-disease control. Smith believes that such policies provide both structure and consistency for a program and that they should go through established channels for congregational approval and be reviewed annually.

Ziebarth (2006) suggests the development of a policy and procedure manual that includes policies on abuse (of children, adults, and the elderly), blood pressure screening guidelines, confidentiality, death in the home, documentation, referral information, infection control, safety, transportation of clients, and the use of volunteers. She also recommends inclusion of personnel information for parish nurses, such as evaluations, personal leaves, terminations, professional liability, job descriptions, and professional development.

Professional Liability

Austin et al. (2004) note that, historically, courts have held nurses who work in alternative settings to the same standards as those who work in hospital settings.

===================*FAST FACTS in a NUTSHELL*

More nurses are named in lawsuits today because:

- Consumers are more knowledgeable about health care and have higher expectations.
- The health care system relies more on nurses and nonphysician providers to contain costs.
- Nurses are more autonomous in their practice.
- The courts are expanding the definition of *liability* and hold all types of medical professionals to higher standards of accountability.

Slutz (2010) cautions that liability insurance for clients and volunteers riding in a personal vehicle of the parish nurse needs careful consideration.

Volunteer Liability

Regarding FCNs' liability when practicing nursing as volunteers, Green (2001) states that the law suggests that if professional nurses render nursing services to a person, even on a free-of-charge and volunteer basis, they could be held liable for negligence. Nurses need to know that even with a charitable intent, volunteer nursing activities can involve professional liability. Employer-provided professional liability insurance provides coverage *only* in the job setting, *not* any other settings.

FCNs practicing as volunteers need personal professional liability coverage. Austin et al. (2004) elaborate that nurses' responsibilities do not change when they are donating nursing services, but their legal status does: It becomes less well defined than when employed. They advise volunteer nurses to observe the same standards of care that they would in their paid positions. Specifically, nurses should have medical orders when indicated, should document the care provided and expected follow-up, and have personal professional liability insurance that provides coverage for unpaid nursing practice.

Slutz (2010) suggests that liability issues be addressed for volunteers as well as for FCNs. She recommends that job descriptions be created for volunteers that clearly describe the expectations and skills for particular volunteer roles and that volunteers be educated on the do's and don'ts of helping others. The Volunteer Protection Act of 1998 provides some protection for volunteers who function in good faith but does not cover organizations for which volunteers provide service.

Professional Liability Insurance

All FCNs should carry personal liability insurance and be covered under the faith community's liability policy as well.

FAST FACTS in a NUTSHELL

Resources Related to Volunteer Liability

- Nonprofit Risk Management Center
  www.nonprofitrisk.org/
- www.nonprofitrisk.org/library/articles/insurance
  052004.shtml
- www.nonprofitexpert.com/volunteers.htm

Resources Related to Liability Insurance

- www.npjobs.com/malpractice/mag.myth.vs.fact.
  shtm
- www.npjobs.com/malpractice/index.shtml
- http:global.marsh.com/index.php
- www.personal-plans.com/anacma/welcome.do
- www.nso.org

Confidentiality and HIPAA

The Health Insurance and Portability and Accountability Act of 2003 (HIPAA) protects all individually identifiable health information in any form. It applies to all health care plans, health clearinghouses, and health care providers who transmit health information. Under HIPAA, only those with a need to know about patient information for the patient's care and only those authorized by the patient may have access to medical records.

Oral communications that FCNs have with patients should not be shared with anyone, including the pastor and the health ministry team, without express permission of the patient. It is good practice for the FCN to ask a patient whether information may be shared with the pastor and, if appropriate, to have that person remembered by name in prayer (and to document this permission).

DOCUMENTATION AND FAITH COMMUNITY NURSING PRACTICE

Parker (2004) believes that documentation is important in faith community nursing as a means of reporting to the congregation and gaining program support. Progress reports, with quantitative data, communicate the volume of and kinds of activities provided by the health ministry. Reporting also enables church staff to evaluate the program and measure its worth to the congregation.

FCNs screen, assess, counsel, educate, and refer people in a variety of settings. While maintaining confidentiality, FCNs must accurately document health-related findings, referrals, and outcomes of care. Patient records provide legal proof of the nature of care. Documentation should be complete, accurate, and timely.

Several formats exist to structure documentation. In the traditional narrative format, FCNs document ongoing assessment data, nursing interventions, and client outcomes in chronological order, but writing narrative notes is time consuming and may be repetitive.

═══════════════════════════*FAST FACTS in a NUTSHELL*

The Problem-Oriented Documentation System: SOAP Notes

S: Subjective client data
O: Objective client data
A: Assessment of subjective complaints and objectives findings
P: Plan

The DIARY Format of Documentation

D: Data
I: Interpretation

Continued

Continued

A: Action
R: Response
Y: Yield

Note: The DIARY documentation format, derived from focus charting (Lampe, 1985), was used in the Parish Nurse Effectiveness Study (Rydholm, 2006).

Regardless of the format chosen to document nursing care, FCNs should do the following when documenting:

- Make sure the client's name is on every page of the record.
- Document symptoms or complaints in the client's own words.
- Document all nursing interventions and the follow-up timeframe.
- Document all of the client's responses to treatment or education.
- Document all health teaching and literature provided to the client.
- Document referrals and follow-up outcomes.
- Sign every entry.

Congregational client records should be stored in a locked filing cabinet or in a secure computer file. When the FCN is employed by a health care system, the system is the legal owner of the medical records. If the FCN is employed by a congregation or is a volunteer, the records belong to the congregation. HIPAA requires that inactive records be stored for 10 years and that records of children be stored until they reach age 21. HIPAA grants patients access to their records. FCNs should document that they have provided copies of records to patients.

Documentation in church settings has experienced some issues. Green (2001) admonishes FCNs to set clear parameters for referral of persons with abnormal screening findings to a physician or an emergency department. She cautions that FCNs could be held liable if they do not provide appropriate follow-up and referral, and have their actions documented.

Parker (2004) studied volunteer FCNs' perceptions of their responsibility to document their activities. Findings indicated that 88% of the 81 participants documented the services provided, 71% noted observations made in assessments, and 78% listed referrals made. Only 48% of respondents reported documenting the outcome(s) of referrals made, only 50% reported having provided a written report to the pastor and/or health ministry team, and 34% reported never providing a written report to the church. Parker voices concern about the findings and believes that improvement is needed for compliance with state practice acts and ANA–HMA standards of practice for faith community nursing. He notes the importance of documenting outcomes of referrals made.

Boss (2004) reports that the application of *Faith Community Nursing: Scope and Standards of Practice* (ANA–HMA, 2005) varies among faith communities, especially in volunteer models. She strongly states that the FCN cannot pick and choose preferred nursing activities at the expense of legally required activities.

SELECTED LEGAL ISSUES AND FAITH COMMUNITY NURSING

Patient's Bill of Rights

The idea of a formal document describing the rights of patients has existed since the 1950s. Over time, hospitals, nursing organizations, hospices, and legal organizations have crafted documents entitled "Patient's Bill of Rights." Minnesota was the first state to enact a patients' bill of rights into law in 1973. At the national level, the U.S.

Commission on Consumer Protection and Quality in the Health Care Industry adopted the Consumer Bill of Rights and Responsibilities in 1998, which applies to the insurance plans offered to federal employees and has been adopted by many other organizations.

KEY AREAS OF THE CONSUMER BILL OF RIGHTS AND RESPONSIBILITIES

- Information for patients
- Choice of providers and plans
- Access to emergency services
- Taking part in treatment decisions
- Respect and nondiscrimination
- Confidentiality of health information
- Complaints and appeals processes
- Consumer responsibilities

Informed Consent

Most nurses are very familiar with the patient right of informed consent. *Informed consent* means that a patient or someone acting on the patient's behalf has enough information to know what risk is involved with a proposed treatment or surgical procedure, what the expected outcome will be, and what the consequences of no action would be. It involves telling the patient what alternatives to the proposed treatment or procedure exist and the risks and benefits associated with each one. The patient must be informed of the name and credentials of the person who will perform the procedure. The patient has the right to refuse consent and to change his or her mind after giving consent.

In the faith community setting, informed consent is required prior to screening procedures. FCNs who provide flu immunization programs must inform patients about the immunization, screen patients for allergies contraindicating the immunization, and provide information about possible side effects.

Usually, the person giving consent for the care of a minor child is a parent or other designated adult, but state laws do vary. Parental consent is required for most medical procedures in most states; however, federal law does allow adolescents to be screened for HIV without parental involvement. Some states permit minors to consent to contraceptive services, and parental consent is not always required to seek prenatal care or treatment for a STD. Every state allows emancipated minors to consent to medical treatment (Tillett, 2005).

Child Abuse, Abuse of the Elderly, and Domestic Violence

In 1973, Congress passed the Child Abuse Prevention and Treatment Act, which requires states to meet certain uniform standards to be eligible for federal assistance for child abuse programs, prevention, and treatment. These include:

- Empowering of social or law enforcement agencies to receive and investigate reports of actual or suspected abuse.
- Granting of legal immunity from liability, for defamation or invasion of privacy, for reporting an incident of actual or suspected abuse.
- Nullification of confidentiality, privacy, and privilege mandates that would otherwise be required of nurse–patient relationships.

All nurses are required to report suspected child abuse. In many states, failure to do so is a crime. Nearly every state has parallel laws regarding abuse of the elderly. Laws regarding domestic violence are less clear. FCNs should be alert to signs and symptoms of domestic violence and know about available community resources for shelter, counseling, emergency services, and law enforcement.

Right to Die

Most states have enacted right-to-die laws that recognize a patient's right to choose death by refusing extraordinary treatment when there is no hope of recovery. Written expression of the patient's wishes may be provided through:

- A *living will,* which is an advance directive document that specifies a person's wishes about medical treatment.
- *Durable power of attorney for health care* is designated by the patient to make medical decisions when the patient is unable to do so.

All states have living will laws that outline the requirements of these documents.

============================*FAST FACTS in a NUTSHELL*

Web resources for advanced directives include:

- End of Life Care Training and courses:
  www.aacn.nche.edu.elnec
- State Advanced Directives forms:
  www.partnershipforcaring.org
- Consumer's Tool Kit:
  www.abanet.org/aging/toolkit/home.html

7

The Ethics of Practicing
Faith Community Nursing

INTRODUCTION

Ethical decisions in faith community nursing are guided by professional elements (ANA Code of Ethics for Nurses, the Public Health Code of Ethics, and the ANA Code for Nurses with Interpretive Statements), and theological and personal elements (Faith Community Nursing: Scope and Standards of Practice, the Ethic of Care, and Christian Ethics).

In this chapter you will learn:

1. Ethical codes in nursing practice and in community faith nursing.
2. Ethical practice in nursing specific to a faith community.

ETHICS IN FAITH COMMUNITY NURSING

Ethics, an area of philosophy, is the systematic study of morality: traditions and beliefs about what is right and wrong. Ethics is concerned with standards of moral conduct and moral judgments. Faith community nursing is the only nursing specialty that is both a practice and a ministry. A ministry within a faith community is bound by and to the teachings, belief system, and values of that community. Ethical decisions in faith community nursing are affected by professional elements (*ANA Code of Ethics for Nurses*, 2002), theological elements, and personal elements. (the person faced with decisions)

ETHICAL CODES

According to Lachman (2009), "A code of ethics is a fundamental document for any profession. It provides a social contract with the society served, as well as ethical and legal guidance to all members of the profession" (p. 55). Professional ethical codes provide guidelines for appropriate ethical decision making and set the standards of conduct for practicing ethically in a specific discipline. The *ANA Code for Nurses with Interpretive Statements* (2002) provides ethical standards for nursing practice, research, and education, and makes the profession's primary goals, values, and obligations explicit.

=====*FAST FACTS in a NUTSHELL*

The Public Health Code of Ethics (2001)

- Consists of 12 principles about the ethical practice of public health.
- Includes the 11 values and beliefs that focus on health, community, and action.
- Focuses on keeping people healthy as the collective and societal nature of public health.
- Addresses the ethical tenets of preventing harm, doing no harm, and promoting good.

FAITH COMMUNITY NURSING: SCOPE AND STANDARDS OF PRACTICE

Professional Performance Standard 12 of *Faith Community Nursing: Scope and Standards of Practice* (American Nurses Association & Health Ministries Association [ANA–HMA], 2005) speaks explicitly to ethics: "The faith community nurse integrates ethical provisions in all areas of practice" (p. 29). The measurement criteria for this standard are that the FCN:

- Uses the *ANA Code of Ethics with Interpretative Statements* to guide practice.
- Acknowledges and respects tenets of faith and spiritual belief system of a patient.
- Delivers care in a manner that preserves and protects patient autonomy, dignity, rights, and spiritual beliefs and practices.
- Maintains patient confidentiality within religious, legal, and regulatory parameters.
- Serves as a patient advocate assisting patients in developing skills for self-advocacy in support of their spiritual beliefs and practices.
- Maintains a therapeutic and professional patient–nurse relationship with appropriate professional role boundaries.
- Demonstrates a commitment to practicing self-care, growing spiritually, managing stress, and remaining connected with both with a centered self and with others.
- Contributes to resolving ethical issues of patients, colleagues, or systems, as evidenced in such activities as participating on ethics committees.
- Reports illegal, incompetent, or impaired practices.
- Participates on multidisciplinary and interdisciplinary teams that address ethical risks, benefits, and outcomes (ANA–HMA, p. 29).

Ethical Practice in a Faith Community

Fowler (1999) states that FCNs face much the same fundamental ethical issues as nurses in other health care settings. Issues of respect for the wishes of congregants, capacity to give consent, privacy and confidentiality, end-of-life decisions, truthfulness and promise keeping, and advocacy and intercession confront nurses in all settings. However, faith community nursing practice gives new meaning and emphasis to ethical practice. The commitment to pray for each other and share a journey of faith is the norm from which ethical actions follow. The discernment of good and evil, right and wrong, is tied to a theological framework as opposed to a secular one. Scripture, prayer, creeds, and confessions are elements of a theological perspective.

Fowler goes on to say that faith community nursing joins the concepts of *vocation* and *covenant community* together with specialized nursing practice: "Its identify is vocational, its intent is ministry, its instrument is nursing, its involvement is covenantal" (p. 187). The vocational aspect of faith community nursing is a call to special work for which one has been given gifts and in which one finds self-identity. The intent is ministry that serves to promote whole health, or *shalom*. The FCN's instrument is nursing, and nursing practice is covenantal in that the nurse is a member of the community in which members are bound together by their belief in God. One's view of faith community nursing is shaped by the community of worship and fellowship, the sacred scriptures, creeds and confessions, and the canon of faith and prayer.

Definitions

FCNs have obligations specific to the profession's practice and goals. These obligations have been interpreted as principles of bioethics: respect for autonomy, nonmaleficence, beneficence, distributive justice, confidentiality, veracity, and fidelity. While these principles have no inherent rank, context and value systems may suggest rankings.

Ethic of Care

While many ethical theories exist, the care-focused feminist approach is particularly congruent with faith community nursing. The ethic of care relates to reciprocal human relationships and connections, preserving personhood, alleviating vulnerability, and is a moral ideal in itself. Gilligan (1982) argues that women, through meeting the needs of children, elderly family members, and people with illness, have developed a language of care that helps create and maintain a thick web of loving human relationships. Tong (2011) believes that care-focused ethical feminists believe people should try to meet one another's genuine needs simply because they are subject to the same vicissitudes of life.

Scholarly work on caring in nursing has been done by many nurse scholars and theorists. Leininger (1984) wrote about caring as the essence of nursing. Watson (1985) focused on caring as a moral imperative. Benner and Wrubel (1989) wrote about the primacy of caring, and Bishop and Scudder (1991) focused on the practice of caring. Current theory in caring science includes Eriksson's (2002), which she describes as ethical in its essence.

Benner addresses the primacy of caring in nursing practice and states that outcomes are not the only issues of care, but that maintaining ties, human connectedness and human concerns, and responding to creation and life as gifts are understood to constitute what it is to be a person. She describes ministering in specific ways to others as profoundly sacred and hopeful (Benner, 1999), ideas that are very congruent with faith community nursing.

Christian Ethics

Ustal (2003) describes the ethic of care from a Christian perspective, emphatically stating that a nurse is the ethic of care and nursing as a ministry is a response to one's faith.

==========*FAST FACTS in a NUTSHELL*

According to Ustal (2003), Christian nurses:

- Recognize that nursing is a calling from God.
- Believe that God has given them a special gift to serve others.
- View nursing as a ministry with commitment to service and a covenantal relationship with the patient, which involves beneficence.
- Experience the ethic of care from God, who promises, "Those who wait for the Lord shall renew their strength, they shall mount up with wings like eagles, they shall run and not be weary, they shall walk and not faint" (Isa. 40:31). (pp. 14–17)

Ustal describes the ethic of care, in brief: to show up, shut up (be fully present, seek the client's story, suspend judgment, stick with him or her), and assure the client that you will help. She encourages nurses to practice the ethic of care in all relationships.

The Judeo-Christian ethic is based on God's holy, unchanging character. Scripture teaches standards of right and wrong, which are based on God's holy, just, and loving character. The Bible outlines principles of justice for society, living with respect and love of God, and the principle of loving and caring for one another in a Christian community.

Ethical Decision Making

Each of the roles of FCNs require ethical decision making. Often, the FCN is called on by faith community members to help them resolve ethical issues. Ethical decision making frameworks use problem solving processes and serve as guides to making decisions that can be morally justified. Decision-making frameworks provide structure and objectivity; they do not, however, provide answers to dilemmas.

=====================================*FAST FACTS in a NUTSHELL*

When faced with an ethical dilemma, the FCN should consider the following:

- What is the issue? What further information is needed for decision making?
- Who will be affected by the decision?
- What are the values of the persons involved?
- What alternatives are available? What are the possible outcomes of each?

Ethics and Health Care

Advances in health care and technology have created new challenges and ethical dilemmas. In nursing practice, ethical decision making is further complicated by sociocultural factors, legal controversies, and consumer involvement in health care. Secular ethics places great emphasis on the principle of autonomy, the right of an individual to choose one's path. However, because faith communities hold values and ethics that are congruent with their theological traditions, reliance on the principle of autonomy may be an insufficient or inappropriate guideline for FCNs.

It is essential that the FCN clearly understand the theological position of the faith community regarding the right to die, organ transplants, blood transfusions, abortion, genetics, and reproductive methods. Denominational Websites provide faith community policy positions about sensitive ethical issues and may serve as a resource to the FCN.

Assessing, Implementing, and Evaluating in Faith Community Ministries

8

Initiating the Faith Community
Nursing Program

INTRODUCTION

*Beginning a new faith community nursing program is
both exciting and challenging. This chapter focuses on
best practices for this endeavor to be a success!*

In this chapter you will learn:

1. The developmental process of initiating a faith community nursing
   program.
2. The process of hiring a FCN.
3. How to work with the ministry team.
4. How to develop resources and professional networks.

BEGINNING STEPS

Brudenell (2003) conducted a study to describe the development and effectiveness of parish nurse programs. A qualitative design, using the grounded theory method, was used to answer the following research questions:

- How do faith communities form a parish nurse program?
- What is the effect of parish nursing programs on health outcomes?

Participants in the study were 13 parish nurses and 8 pastors, representing 13 congregations with parish nurse programs; 2 hospital chaplains, and 2 parish nurse coordinators ($N = 24$). Eight denominations were represented and church membership ranged from 80 to 2,500. Rural, suburban, and urban congregations were included. The findings of this study indicate that the formation of a parish nurse programs is a developmental process comprised of four phases:

- A preliminary phase of finding out or thinking about parish nursing
- Knowing the faith community
- Being accepted as part of the congregation's ministry
- Becoming an ongoing ministry that distinguishes a congregation

FCNs come to their positions in a variety of ways. Some nurses are approached by their minister to consider assuming the role for their congregation. Others answer an ad for a position or initiate the idea of starting a parish nurse program with the faith community leader. For many nurses, faith community nursing is an opportunity to blend their spiritual and professional life together in a unique way. The FCN working in the faith community has the opportunity to work with individuals and families for long time periods and to focus on holistic health in ways rarely possible in other nursing settings.

Patterson (2003) relates parish nursing to Christian diaconal ministry. *Diakonia* is the Greek word for "service." The early Christian Church recognized service to others on behalf of the church as a ministry. Diaconal ministry is a fusion of care for the body and soul in the context of community. Christian theological frameworks support diaconal ministries that follow the example set by Christ as an opportunity to serve as a witness for Him, and by serving those in need, provide service to Christ. According to Patterson, diaconal ministries historically were faith-based responses to human needs in times when governments had no organized response. FCNs of all faith traditions are following sacred footsteps, doing holy work.

═══════════════════════*FAST FACTS in a NUTSHELL*

The Evangelical Lutheran Church in America (2010) lists diaconal ministers' characteristics:

- Be rooted in the Word of God.
- Be trained to carry out a particular service.
- Be committed and prepared to equip the baptized for ministry in the world and in the Church.
- Give particular attention to ministries at the boundaries between the Church and the world.
- Exemplify a life of Christ-like service addressing all forms of human need.
- Be grounded in community.

Brudenell (2003) describes the preliminary phase of beginning a parish nurse program as "thinking about parish nursing," in which both pastors and nurses recounted how they first heard about a health and spirituality program. Several pastors had heard about parish nursing programs at national conferences and knew their denominations had well-established health information and ministry programs. Three pastor-participants in the study recounted positive benefits to their congregations achieved with parish nurses.

Some pastors viewed health ministry as another way to connect congregational members with the health care system as well as to community resources. Having a health professional available and willing was a deciding factor in developing a health ministry.

Catanzaro, Meador, Koenig, Kuchibhatia, and Clipp (2007) surveyed 349 pastors from over 80 Christian denominations and found that with limited resources, church health ministries provided significant health promotion, disease prevention, and support services to their congregations. The authors found that the long-term trusting relationships that exist between congregants and those who minister to them make religious congregations ideally suited to provide cost-effective, community-based health promotion and disease prevention services, as well as health-supporting services to community-dwelling elderly persons with chronic diseases.

Chase-Ziolek (2003) raises the issue of terminology noting that *health ministry* serves as the umbrella term most commonly used to describe a church's role in health, with parish nursing being one aspect of health ministry. As *health ministry* joins two concepts, health and ministry, it has appeal to both health and ministry professionals. Chase-Ziolek, however, believes that the term *ministries of health* more clearly defines the work because it provides the perspective of how ministries of health fit into a congregation's culture and understanding, rather than simply bringing health services to the church.

Historically, the health care industry has been inconsistent about support for health ministries, and institutionally sponsored health ministries are vulnerable to budget cuts. However, when health promotion and disease prevention are understood as essential ministries, the congregation will find a means to provide support for it.

Garity and Ryan (2002) believe an advisory board can help parish nurses and congregations interested in starting a parish nurse program to avoid common pitfalls.

==*FAST FACTS in a NUTSHELL*

Common Pitfalls to Avoid in Parish Nursing Programs
(Meyer, 1996):

- Having no strategy
- Poor planning
- Weak organization
- Ineffective leadership
- Lack of control

Garity and Ryan advise having an advisory board of carefully recruited professionals with expertise in administration, nursing, education, social work, and theology. The purposes of the advisory board are to shape a mission for the program, establish policies and program guidelines, and provide mentoring to the parish nurse coordinator. They report positive program outcomes using this approach.

Patterson (2003), on the other hand, uses the term *health cabinet,* also a group of five to seven health professionals who provide direction and assistance to the health ministry of a congregation in the following areas:

- *Theological reflection.* The health cabinet should spend time reflecting on the Biblical mandates to teach and heal and holistically care for one's neighbor.
- *Personnel.* The health cabinet recommends the type of parish nurse program to be offered (full- or part-time) and compensation, if any, for a parish nurse. The health cabinet recruits, hires the FCN, and conducts annual performance reviews.
- *Strategic planning.* The health cabinet meets with the parish nurse to help assess the congregation's health needs and help plan programs to meet those needs.
- *Volunteers.* The health cabinet can help match members' gifts and talents with the needs of the health ministry.
- *Fundraising.* The health cabinet can help with fundraising events and grant proposal writing.

HIRING A FAITH COMMUNITY NURSE

Great diversity exists in faith communities' governance structures and financial resources. A starting point is the development of an advisory board or health cabinet. A committee of people endorsing the establishment of a health ministry provides more credibility than a perception of the parish nurse program as being an individual ministry (Metzger, 2006). Once a health cabinet is in place, the members must become informed about possibilities for the ministry through Web-based research, using consultants, and visiting programs at other faith communities. The International Parish Nurse Resource Center (IPNRC) Website provides a wealth of information about starting a parish nurse program.

The first step in the hiring process of a FCN is the development of a job description which outlines the functions and roles that the nurse will (or will not) provide for the members of the faith community. If community outreach is also expected, this should be clearly stated. It is important to consider whether the expectations are in line with the hours to be worked. Figure 8.1 provides the INPRC's sample job description for a parish nurse. Note that the job description is based on Westburg's seven parish nurse roles. It is very thorough and can be modified to meet the needs and expectations of a congregation.

The IPNRC recommends that a parish nurse have a BSN with clinical experience in medical-surgical nursing and community health nursing. The ability to do a community assessment and plan care for populations are key competencies needed for parish nursing. Theological or clinical pastoral education is an asset as well.

Metzger (2006) states that spiritual leadership experiences and the ability to function as part of a team are special job characteristics related to faith community nursing. However, the actual minimum requirement is to be an RN.

The findings of a recent study by Ziebarth and Miller (2010) identify deficiencies in parish nurse training that

Figure 8.1   Job Description for the Ministry of Parish Nursing Practice

This position is designed to provide whole person health promotion disease prevention services with an emphasis on spiritual care. The major accountabilities and job activities of the parish nurse role are integrator of faith and health, health educator, personal health counselor, referral agent, developer of support groups, trainer of volunteers and health advocate.

I. Accountabilities

Integrator of faith and health
- Assesses congregation's assets and needs incorporating an understanding of the relationship between faith and health.
- Participates as a staff member of the congregation, attending all meetings of the staff of the congregation.
- Identifies opportunities to enhance the understanding of the relationship of faith and health within the congregation.
- Fosters, promotes, and provides opportunities for spiritual care to be discussed and integrated into the parish nurse role documenting spiritual care of groups and individuals.
- Participates in the planning and providing of prayer and worship life of the congregation.
- Teaches and models the integration of faith and health into daily life.

Personal health counselor
- Provides individual health counseling related to health maintenance, disease prevention or illness patterns.

Continued

Figure 8.1   *Continued*

- Encourages the client through presence and spiritual support to express their faith beliefs and utilize them regularly especially in time of crisis and despair.
- Documents client assessment, nursing diagnosis, interventions and outcomes while maintaining confidential client record in accordance with the policy on documentation.
- Make visits to clients as needed providing health counseling, education and spiritual presence/support.
- Promotes stewardship of the body emphasizing self care of the whole person.
- Collaborates with pastoral staff to plan for health education programming.
- Communicates with other health professionals as needed to meet the health needs of clients.

Health educator
- Utilizes information from asset and needs assessments of the congregation and surrounding community in planning for education programs.
- Prepares, develops and/or coordinates educational programs based on identified needs for healthier lifestyles, early illness detection and health resources.
- Maintains records of educational programs, including objectives, content, evaluation, attendance and budget.
- Documents individual educational assessment diagnosis, interventions and outcomes.
- Provides the pastor, health committee of the congregation, and other designated parties a summary

Continued

Figure 8.1   *Continued*

evaluation of educational programs noting attendance and response of participants.
- Networks with appropriate resources in the community to secure educational program resources.
- Provides consultation and acts as a health resource
to other staff of the congregation.

Trainer of volunteers
- Identifies and recruits professional and lay
volunteers who can be available to respond
to the health related needs of members of the
congregation.
- Facilitates and when appropriate, trains individuals to assume volunteer responsibilities to meet
identified needs of the congregation.
- Works with staff, health committee or others
focusing on the integration of health into the life
of the congregation.

Developer of support groups
- Develops and/or facilitates support groups based
on identified needs and resources.
- Identifies available support groups in the community that could resource the congregation.
- Refers and documents client participation in designated support groups.

Referral agent
- Provides and documents referrals to health care
services and resources within the congregation
and external community.
- Collaborates with community leaders and agencies to facilitate effective working relationships
while identifying new health resources.

Continued

Figure 8.1 *Continued*

- Develops community contacts in order to secure resources and services to meet the needs of members of the congregation.
- Networks with other parish nurses and professionals.

Health advocate
- Encourages clients to avail themselves of services, which will enhance their overall well-being, assisting the clients in identifying values, and choices, which encourage them to be more responsible for their health status.
- Assists client and client families in making decisions regarding their health, medical services,treatments and care facilities as well as documenting assessments, diagnosis, interventions and outcomes.
- Identifies, communicates, and works cooperatively with community leaders, elected officials, and agencies to meet health needs of members of the congregation and surrounding community.

II. Job Activities

Management
- Prepares an operating budget for program development as needed.
- Develops reports regarding parish nurse activities as needed.
- Collaborates with others in developing and managing grant projects.
- Coordinates all parish nurse programming in the congregation.

Continued

Figure 8.1 *Continued*

Professional development, education and research
- Participates in continuing education programs to meet identified professional learning needs.
- Participates in regular personal spiritual formation.
- Acts as a preceptor to students from schools of nursing, seminaries and other disciplines as requested.
- Develops and/or participates in research related to parish nursing.
- Develops and submits articles for publication on experiences in parish nursing.

III. Job Requirements

	Competent Level Qualifications	*Minimum Level Qualifications*
Skills	Organizing skill Basic computer skills Excellent communication skills Ability to develop reports	Excellent communication skills Organizing skills
Education and experience	BSN required 5+ years experience in med-surg Community health nursing experience desirable Ability to do community assessments Ability to do health counseling	BS preferred 5 years clinical nursing experience Assessment skills

Continued

Figure 8.1   *Continued*

Professional preparation	Current license as a registered nurse in the state the congregation is located. Completion of a basic preparation course in parish nursing based on the standardized core curriculum endorsed through the International Parish Nurse Resource Center.	Current license as a registered nurse in the state the congregation is located.
Special job characteristics	Spiritual leadership as evidenced by experience in congregational ministries, lay leadership, theological education and other related spiritual development. Substantial weekend and evening work.	Works well independently and yet can function well as part of a work team. Has a good understanding of spirituality and religiosity.

© 2010 Deaconess Parish Nurse Ministries, LLC. Used with permission.

lead to feelings of inadequacy in areas such as spirituality and community nursing knowledge. Participants reported that lectures, peer sharing activities, and peer and church leader mentoring were helpful in successful role transition. Challenges included the brevity of courses about parish nursing, content being too "packed in," and the inclusion of inexperienced student nurses in courses. Challenges to role transition were lack of time to attend peer support (parish nurse) meetings and to practice the roles, lack of a mentor, and congregational lack of knowledge about parish nursing roles. It may be premature to consider certification of an advanced practice parish nurse until attention is given to basic educational standards.

An understanding of the state's nurse practice act and *Faith Community Nursing: Scope and Standards of Practice* is needed to direct the FCN's legal scope of practice. Members of the congregation need to be educated about the role of the FCN. While many would like to have a faith-based home health nurse to provide physical care and treatment, these are not appropriate functions for the FCN. The role of the FCN emphasizes whole person health and wellness with a focus on prevention and health.

Once the decision is made to initiate a faith community nursing program, the hiring of the FCN needs to be addressed, including the issue of hiring from within or outside the congregation. Hiring an insider has the advantage of the nurse knowing the formal and informal structures of the faith community, its leadership, and spiritual traditions. The challenge for an insider nurse is the congregation accepting him or her in the new role.

Patterson (2003) recommends hiring a nurse from outside the faith community because he or she has no preconceived ideas about the faith community or historical knowledge, and therefore has more objectivity. If the decision is made to hire outside of the congregation, the health cabinet needs to advertise the position, consider only applicants with the required credentials, and interview the top three candidates before making a recommendation to the senior pastor, who will then make the job offer.

If the faith community is paying the parish nurse, a decision is needed about benefits, ncluding health, life, and disability insurance; retirement savings; tuition reimbursement; sick leave; and vacation time. Obviously, what benefits can be offered depend on the financial resources of the faith community. The congregation should carry institutional liability insurance, and the FCN should have person professional liability coverage as well.

THE FCN AND THE PASTOR

All the literature about parish nursing supports the importance of a collegial relationship between the pastoral ministry staff and the parish nurse. Support from the leadership and a good working relationship are essential to success in any organizational effort. Also essential is the FCN's ability to clearly understand and participate in both the theological and pastoral cultures of the faith community, The relationship between the pastor and FCN must be built on respect, trust, and support, with the FCN keeping the pastoral staff well informed and consulting with them as needed.

Blanchfield and McLaughlin (2006) remind us that the roles of the professional staff in faith communities are to call, unite, empower, and support all members of the congregation to use their gifts to continue the work of the Lord and build His Kingdom. The parish nurse becomes the instrument of empowering people of good will to be alert to and respond to the needs of those who are sick, aged, or infirm.

Metzger (2006) advises that the FCN must understand the administrative structure of the congregation and be aware of its formal and informal leaders, as well as the pastor's passions and influences. The pastoral staff and FCN must agree on program's goals, and the pastoral staff introduces the FCN into the committee structures of the church. If the pastoral staff is supportive, the committee structures will likely be also and will share the idea of a new faith community nursing program with others.

INITIATING THE MINISTRY OF
FAITH COMMUNITY NURSING

The first step to initiating a new faith community nursing program is to educate the congregation about the roles and functions of the FCN. This can be accomplished by clear explanations, printed information (in bulletins, in a brochure, and on bulletin boards), and addressing the congregation during worship service. For some faith communities, an installation service is held to welcome the nurse into the ministry of the congregation. Such a service indicates the values placed on the ministry as well as the support of pastoral leadership. Members of the health cabinet should also act as ambassadors for the parish nurse program within the congregation.

Essential to success of a new program is that goals remain simple and clear, it is started modestly, and stays focused on immediate goals and objectives. Small programs with early success provide the foundation upon which faith community nursing is built.

Brudenell describes the second phase of establishing a faith community nursing program as "knowing the faith community." Pastors and nurses must know their congregations and what they need and want for their health ministry, which is achieved by conducting a congregational needs assessment (to be discussed in depth in Chapter 9). Based on data collected in the assessment process, programs are planned. It is important to assure the congregation members that programs will be planned based on their areas of interest.

The research literature shows that different faith communities place higher values on different FCN roles. Some prefer the FCN to focus on more traditional nursing roles of health promoter, educator, and risk assessor, whereas others place a higher value on the role of integrator of faith and health. The actual working time will also determine which and how many role functions the FCN can realistically and successfully perform.

Brudenell (2003) identifies the third phase of establishing a parish nurse program as "being accepted as a faith community ministry." This occurs over time as congregation members learn about and interact with the parish nurse. Brudenell states that another indicator of this phase is the growing independence of the health of the health ministry team. Pastors and nurses involved in this study spoke of "being present" or "visible," talking, praying, and being involved in the community as being key to being accepted as a caring community member, as were mutual valuing and responding with caring.

Volunteers are the backbone of a health ministry program and can help it expand its services. Parker believes that volunteers are uplifted in their own personal faith journey as a result of volunteering and describes a three-step process to motivate volunteers: inviting, igniting, and uniting. Wuthnow (2004) reports that members of religious communities are twice as likely to be involved in volunteer activities as nonmembers. He states that doing volunteer work is reinforced by what he calls *spiritual practice,* which involves intentional activity concerned with strengthening one's relationship with God.

Hinton suggests that, to protect the faith community and the FCN, all volunteers should consent to a background check; have clear guidelines, orientation, and training; and be adequately supervised. She also suggests that clear policies be in place for the dismissal of volunteers and that the total number of volunteer hours provided to a health ministry program be included in the FCN's annual report. The Independent Sector (2010) estimated the average value of volunteer time in the United States in 2009 at $20.85/hour. The FCN can use this figure to determine the value of time given to the health ministry.

=====*FAST FACTS in a NUTSHELL*

Resources About Volunteers

Hurley, J., & Mohnkern, S. Mobilize support groups to meet congregational needs. *Journal of Christian Nursing,* 2004; 21(4): 34–39.

Miller, K. No more don't ask, don't tell. *Leadership Journal.net.* 2010.

http://www.christianitytodya.com/le/2010/spring/nomoredontask.html?start=1

Continued

Continued

Locker, D. (2010). *The Volunteer Book: A Guide for Churches and Nonprofits*. Kansas City, MO: Beacon Hill.
http://www.stephenministries.org
http://befrienderministy.org

Brudenell's final phase of establishing a faith community nursing program is "parish nursing as an ongoing ministry." At that point, a faith community nursing program is recognized by the congregation as established and essential. A program that has reached this phase is characterized by continuous outreach to others both within and outside the congregation. Working relationships of the pastor, parish nurse, health ministry team, church staff, congregants, and community are evident and positive.

════════════════════════ *FAST FACTS in a NUTSHELL*

Resources Needed for a FCN

- A desk, phone, answering machine, and lockable file cabinet for client records
- Ideally, a laptop computer in which to keep all client records
- Private office space for consultation and counseling
- Storage space supplies and health education materials
- An automobile and, ideally, a GPS system

As the FCN works in an independent role, attention to scope of practice is essential. The FCN must establish a method of record keeping and documentation of all activities, and also comply with health privacy laws. Figure 8.2 provides the IPNRC's sample budget.

Figure 8.2   Sample Parish Nursing Budget

A line item budget is an excellent way to integrate the ministry of parish nursing practice into the financial life of the congregation. The budget below is a suggestion for parish nurses in congregations. The amount of money necessary for each item depends on many factors. Some considerations are the overall budget of the congregation, the number of educational programs that will be offered, the size of the congregation, and the overall goals and objectives identified for the parish nurse for the budget year.

Revenue
A. Gifts, donations, memorials
B. Fundraisers
C. Grants

Expenses
A. Salary/Stipend
B. Benefits
C. Liability insurance

Other Expenses
A. Equipment
B. Blood pressure equipment (3 sizes of cuffs)
C. Stethoscope
D. Scale
E. Office space with phone/answering machine
F. Computer/printer
G. File cabinets, locked and preferably fireproof
H. Desk, chair, bookshelves
I. Educational materials
J. Travel

Continued

Figure 8.2   *Continued*

K. Postage
L. Photocopying/printing
M. Honorarium for speakers
N. Continuing Education and professional asso-
   ciation memberships
O. Lodging
P. Meals

Professional Networks

Recent research documents the importance of peer support and mentorship for new FCNs. Often, a FCN is the
only health professional on the faith community staff. It is
strongly suggested that FCNs participate in a regional parish nurse or health ministry organization. Faith community
nursing networks provide insider information, resources,
and cost sharing.

Daloz (1999) describes mentoring as a journey on which
the mentor is a trusted guide. She identifies three primary
roles of a mentor:

• To provide support
• To challenge
• To provide vision

Daloz theorizes that if a person is constantly exposed to
high challenge without support, burnout is likely. If a person experiences little support and little challenge, stasis and
apathy occur. If a person has great support but little challenge, the person is comfortable but not a high performer.
Daloz (1999) posits that the most desirable situation offers
great support and high challenge, a blend that leads to confidence and vision.

Nease (2010) believes that coaching is similar to mentoring but does not require the same depth of relationship. A coach focuses on "how to." Nease goes on to explain that Jesus demonstrated a mentoring style worth emulating. He took 12 common men with potential and mentored them from novice to expert over a 3-year period. He developed close interpersonal relationships with and between them and fostered their holistic development by using common elements to simplify concepts (the mustard seed), using parables to teach, answering questions with questions to encourage thinking beyond the simple, and demonstrating forgiveness and respect while holding them accountable.

Nease identifies the role of the Apostle Paul as that of a coach. He is credited with authoring 13 books of the New Testament, including letters to new churches, new church leaders, and Christians struggling with faith. Paul wrote; "I long to see you so that I may impart to you some spiritual gift to make you strong—that is, that you and I may be mutually encouraged by each other's faith" (Romans 1:11–12). Mutual encouragement is an essence of coaching. Nease states that, in keeping with Dolaz's model, both Jesus and Paul used support and challenge to inspire and develop new vision for their protégés. Nease encourages nurses to "Mentor like Jesus, coach like Paul." This is excellent advice for faith community nurses, both novice and expert.

9

Assessing the Faith Community

INTRODUCTION

Community assessment is the process of looking at a community's characteristics from an analytical point of view to identify its strengths and weaknesses or assets and liabilities. Standard 1 of Faith Community Nursing: Scope and Standards of Practice (ANA–HMA, 2005) focuses on assessment: "The faith community nurse collects comprehensive data pertinent to the patient's holistic health or the situation" (p. 11). When health is viewed from a holistic perspective, a person is seen as an integrated whole, with the whole being greater than and different from the sum of the parts. Holistic nursing supports the connectedness of mind, body, and spirit.

In this chapter you will learn:

1. How to conduct a faith community walk-about assessment.
2. How to conduct a faith community assessment.
3. How to analyze data.

CONCEPTS OF COMMUNITY

In the community assessment process, the faith community is viewed as the client. The faith community is defined as "an organization of groups, families, and individuals who share common values, beliefs, and religious doctrine, and faith practices that influence their lives, such as church, synagogue, or mosques, and that functions as a patient system" (ANA–HMA, 2005, p. 36.) From a systems perspective, the *whole* of the faith community is composed of the sum of the persons, environment, structures, values, and practices of the faith community, with the *whole* being more than and different from the sum of the parts. Because of the interrelatedness of the community, each part of the community affects and is affected by changes in every other part. According to Clark (2000), all faith communities demonstrate characteristics of faith, spirituality, theology, and religion that can be identified and assessed. She describes faith as "being in relationship with," spirituality as "an experience of being in relationship with," theology as "reflections of being in relationship with," and religion as "a community within which to share reflection and celebration around experiences of being in relationship with."

Definitions of *community* are plentiful in the literature. Carroll (2004) states that the following three dimensions are core to any definition of *community:*

- *Status:* information about morbidity and mortality, life expectancy, crime rates, and education.
- *Structure:* the socioeconomic levels, age ranges, gender, and ethnic distributions as well as resources available.
- *Process:* how the community operates; how it functions as a whole to solve problems (p. 52).

Carroll also states that the process dimension of a community includes the concepts of community *competence* and *capacity. Competence* refers to the community's ability to effectively identify needs, achieve working consensus on issues, agree on ways to implement goals, and work together to implement desired actions. Capacity refers to the community's ability to resolve a particular issue or to do a particular job. Community capacity builds on community competence.

═══════════════════════ *FAST FACTS in a NUTSHELL*

Blum (1974) describes several types of communities:

- Face-to-face community
- Neighborhood community
- Community of identifiable need
- Community of problem ecology
- Community of concern
- Community of viability
- Community political jurisdiction
- Community of solution
- Resource community
- Community of special interest

A faith community is always one of special interests and may often be one of solutions for its members. The mission(s) of the faith community may steer a focus of assessment. For example, if there is a strong commitment to serve the youth of a community, this focus would steer the assessment process.

Shuster and Goeppinger (2008) define *community* as "a locality-based entity, composed of systems of formal organizations reflecting society's institutions, informal groups, and aggregates" (p. 343). Personal, geographic, and functional components of community are interrelated. Although a faith community certainly has formal and informal structures, whether it purpsely reflects societal institutions depends on the faith tradition. Many faith traditions, by intent, have value systems that differ from societal institutions.

Ervin (2002) discusses the concept of "community as a relational experience." *Community* is defined as the everyday life experience of living and "being in" community. The experience of "being in" community is having a sense of connection, history, safe places to be, collective memories, hopes, and dreams. It is about the experience of having overlapping lives and interrelationships, and shared emotional connections. The faith community is very much a relational community, but also a community with structure and function. Extended families and religious orders are also relational communities.

Anderson (1990) defines a *faith community* as an assembly of people whose beliefs about God combine with a common identity, shared history, regular worship, and common values to effect personal and social transformation.

===*FAST FACTS in a NUTSHELL*

McKnight (1987) identifies characteristics of faith community associations as:

- Being interdependent: To weaken one part of a community is to weaken the whole community.
- Being structured around the recognition of fallibility rather than the ideal; thus there is room for many leaders.
- Having the capacity to respond quickly because they do not have to move issues through an institutional or corporate structure before taking action.
- Allowing for the flowering of creative solutions.
- Being small, face-to face groups, so relationships are individualized.
- Providing care that represents consent versus control. (p. 56)

The preceding discussions about the concept of community reinforce the idea that faith communities serve as places of holistic health promotion. Health ministry is a seamless garment, demonstrating that faith, health, and wholeness are one. Health ministries are actualized by building caring communities that nurture each person in body, mind, and spirit; by promoting good stewardship of one's body; and by working for a just, equal, and effective system of health care (Health Ministries Association USA, 2004).

ASSESSMENT OF THE FAITH COMMUNITY

The purposes of assessing a faith community include:

• Describing the attributes of the membership.
• Learning its gifts and strengths.
• Identifying its health and spiritual needs.
• Identifying its health risk factors.
• Identifying its needs and interests in health-related services and programs.

How a faith community defines its mission influences what, how much, and when various health assessments are conducted. Large faith communities with established health ministries or health ministry cabinets have a structure in place for a committee to participate in the data collection and analysis aspects of the process. Small faith communities operating with a full-time worship leader and a part-time FCN may need volunteers to help with the assessment process. Ideally, the entire faith community participates in the assessment, and both quantitative and qualitative data are collected and analyzed (Hickman, 2006).

WALK-ABOUT ASSESSMENT

A walk-about is a good starting point for assessment. A walk-about is a mini-assessment of a community performed by walking around and observing the setting. It is helpful to first do a walk-about alone, then again with a person familiar with the faith community. The FCN will collect observational data about the setting and structure of the congregational meeting place (church, temple, mosque), immediate neighborhood, services offered to the membership, and size and nature of the clerical and lay staff (Figure 9.1). The FCN also

Figure 9.1   How to Conduct a Walk-About
                  Assessment

While observing the faith community in action, the
FCN should consider these questions:

Place
- What is this place called?
- About how many people can the worship area
  accommodate?
- Is the structure accessible to people with
  disabilities?
- Are there spaces that can be used for religious and
  health educational activities?
- Are there childcare areas?
- Are there private spaces for staff offices? Are there
  computers and telephones?
- What types of messages are conveyed through
  bulletin boards, banners, or signs?
- Is there a library? A kitchen?
- Is parking available? Is it adequate?
- Is the place of worship accessible by public
  transportation?
- What is the surrounding neighborhood like?
  Are properties well maintained? Are people
  about?
- Do you feel safe walking in this neighborhood in
  the daytime? In the evening?
- Do you feel welcome in this place?

Member Services
- How many worship services are held each week?
- Are worship services attended by the majority of
  the membership?

Continued

Figure 9.1   *Continued*

- Is religious education provided for children? For adults?
- Is childcare available during services?
- What ministries does the faith community provide? Music? Youth? Outreach?
- Are certain age groups over- or under-represented?
- Are there volunteers for services such as childcare and/or serving on committees?

will observe and participate in worship services and other congregational activities.

GATHERING DEMOGRAPHIC DATA

Once the FCN has reviewed information from the walk-about, the next logical step in the assessment process is to review available data about the membership's characteristics. Many congregations keep a computerized database that usually includes names, addresses, telephone numbers, e-mail addresses, and birthdates of members. It may also include an inventory of the talents of the members and their interests in areas of community participation. If this information is available to the FCN, it provides a wonderful starting point for a faith community assessment. If not, the FCN will need to collect these data and organize them carefully.

Demographic data about the membership help the FCN know how to plan for health education programs and how to determine and prioritize needed services. The educational level of the congregation, the cultural diversity (or not), and the use of languages other than English are all important data to collect and analyze. Another area of assessment is the administrative structure of the faith community.

=== *FAST FACTS in a NUTSHELL*

Questions to Ask About the Administrative Structure of the Faith Community

- Who are considered to be leaders in the faith community?
- Who comprises the ministry staff, and what is the hierarchy?
- What are areas of responsibility for each staff member? Do any areas overlap?
- What is the governing body of the faith community? Is it elected by the membership or appointed by the clergy?
- How are decisions made in the faith community? Who must be consulted to approve plans and programs?
- Do both men and women serve in all roles, or are roles gender proscribed?
- Is there a committee structure? Does it include a health ministry? What services does it provide?
- Who develops and manages the faith community budget?
- Are human and financial resources adequate to meet community needs? (Hickman, 2006)

If the faith community has a committee, the FCN can meet with each group to provide information and solicit support for an evolving faith community nursing ministry. The committee structure is an important communication tool for the FCN to explain the possible programs and services a health ministry can provide.

GATHERING DATA THROUGH FOCUS GROUPS

Focus groups are one means of gathering aggregate data about the faith community. They can be existing committees or groups convened specifically to discuss health ministry issues. Clark et al. (2003) suggest that focus groups provide an effective means of incorporating the perspectives of "hidden" populations in a community. Information about what specific kinds of health programs and services that the congregation wants and is willing to participate provides direction to the faith community ministry. Swinney, Anson-Wonkka, Maki, and Corneau (2001) suggest the following questions to guide focus groups discussions:

- What are some things about your health or that of your family that concern you?
- When you are not feeling well, with whom do you usually speak?
- Do you believe the church has a role in helping to meet the health needs of church members? In your opinion, how important is this?
- What types of services would you like to see the church and the FCN work together to establish to help you to better meet your health needs?

Focus groups can provide the FCN with rich information, and the group process introduces the FCN to members in a relational way. A negative aspect of focus groups is that they are time-consuming and provide contact with relatively small numbers of people. Another method of data collection is one-on-one interviews with opinion leaders in the congregation. Like focus groups, individual interviews are time consuming, but they may create allies and advocates for the FCN and provide insider information.

GATHERING DATA USING PAPER-AND-PENCIL SURVEYS

Paper-and-pencil surveys are another method to collect data about the health interests and needs of the faith community. Surveys can be a time-saving approach that allow the FCN to reach all members of the community. Respondents can remain anonymous, which may increase participation. A drawback to surveys is that people can choose not to complete them. Providing an opportunity to complete a survey within the framework of a worship service, with a drop-off box in the back of the church, facilitates completion and return of the survey instrument. As many members as possible should be reached.

Many congregational questionnaires can be modified to meet more specific needs of faith communities and are available in the literature (Figures 9.2 and 9.3). In customizing a survey form, ask only for information that will be used to plan health programs for the community. Be sensitive to what community members may consider private information

---

Figure 9.2   Short Congregational Health Survey

**Dear (Congregant, Parishioner,
Sisters and Brothers)**

Please assist us in planning health programs for our congregation by responding to the following questions. There is no need to sign your name.

Please put an X by your answer.
I have interest in participating in the following types of health screening programs:
_____   Blood pressure (hypertension screening)
_____   Blood sugar (diabetes screening)
_____   Stroke risk assessment

I am interested in learning more about:
_____   Adolescent   _____   Exercise
            health issues   and health

_____   Alternative   _____   Heart
            therapies   disease

Continued

Figure 9.2   *Continued*

_____	Hypertension	_____	Stroke prevention
_____	Alzheimer's disease	_____	Eating disorders
_____	Arthritis	_____	Anxiety disorders
_____	CPR	_____	Cancer
_____	Smoking cessation	_____	Weight control
_____	Women's health issues	_____	Men's health issues
_____	Grief and loss	_____	Sleep disorders
_____	Respiratory disorders	_____	Diabetes
_____	Depression	_____	Menopause

Which day of the week and time would you be interested in attending a program?

_____	Monday	_____	Tuesday
_____	Wednesday	_____	Thursday
_____	Friday	_____	Saturday
_____	Sunday		
_____	Morning	_____	Afternoon
_____	Evening		

and consider both legal and ethical aspects of personal information and confidentiality.

When customizing a survey instrument, give members the opportunity to report positive aspects of personal behaviors related to their health. Asking people what they would

Figure 9.3   Long Congregational Health Survey

What do you do to keep yourself as healthy as possible?

_____

Please mark all of the health-related activities in which you have high interest:

Participate in a health
Sabbath service   _____

Participate in a Health
Awareness Week   _____

Health fair   _____

Exercise program   _____

Weight-control program   _____

Smoking-cessation program   _____

Study groups on health issues   _____

Services of prayer and healing   _____

Parenting skills classes   _____

Health issues for women   _____

Health issues for teens   _____

Health issues for men   _____

Illness screenings   _____

Conflict-management classes   _____

Support groups   _____

Issues of aging   _____

Advance directives/Living wills   _____

Grief and loss   _____

Depression   _____

Other:

Continued

Figure 9.3 *Continued*

Do you need information on any specific health or medical topic or issue?

• Please indicate your preferred day and time for health programming:
_____ After worship services
_____ Evenings
_____ Day of the week

Are you interested in becoming a part of the health ministry of the congregation?

| _____ Provide transportation | _____ Home or hospital visitor |
| _____ Health educator | _____ Assist parish nurse |

Thank you for your participation! Have a blessed day!

like to know more about is much more positive than asking them to identify areas of weakness. Providing checklists of potential topics for programs is helpful for respondents to identify interest areas of personal interest. Try to find out the days and times that members are available to attend health programs.

STRATEGIES FOR ORGANIZING DATA

Data collected from all sources should be recorded in an organized and retrievable manner. A computerized database or spreadsheet program is an efficient method for recording data, but if a computer is not available, a 3-ring binder will work as well. Do consider the level of security required to protect the information collected.

Mayhugh and Martens (2001) report that 80% of their respondents preferred health education programs with information about staying well and with health screening. Over half the respondents wanted the FCN to visit members who were terminally ill, or in a nursing home, or who had recently been released from the hospital. Gottlieb and Allen (1997) identified 8 categories of health-related issues about which people seek nursing expertise:

- Family experiences change in size, composition, roles, and relationships.
- Learn to function in the health care system
- Interact with environmental conditions to develop health-promoting behaviors
- Experience biophysiological changes related to growth and development (puberty, menopause)
- Need to learn to cope with chronic illness in a healthful way
- Encounter episodes of acute illness or injury
- Adapt to changing economic conditions
- Try to maintain interpersonal relationships and/or resolve conflict within a family

These themes can be used to construct a faith community assessment tool.

ANALYSIS OF FAITH COMMUNITY DATA

Once assessment data have been collected, the FCN reviews it to ascertain the descriptive elements about the congregation and to identify common threads in areas of interest for health programs. Data can also be analyzed in terms of community assets and deficits. High-priority items are program or service requests identified by the largest number of respondents and also those to which the FCN and the health ministry can most readily and appropriately respond. Planning for early successes is the best way to introduce new programs. Successes provide positive credibility and publicity to the faith community nursing program. When data analysis yields information outside the scope of nursing, the FCN can refer the issue or problem to the appropriate person.

════════════════FAST FACTS in a NUTSHELL

The Community Tool Box (http://ctb.ku.edu/tool/assess-community/index.jsp) provides resources and guidance on conducting community assessment, with a focus on building healthy communities. "Tools" includes an entire section on community assessment.

10

Education for Health

INTRODUCTION

The health educator role of the FCN has been extensively developed in practice. In this role, the FCN empowers the individual, family, or congregation to incorporate health and healing practices from a faith perspective to achieve positive health outcomes. Faith community nursing practice respects the dignity of the person and views stewardship of the body and personal health as a responsibility to God and respect for His creation.

In this chapter you will learn about:

1. Using health education models for behavioral change.
2. Assessing literacy levels.
3. Using a variety of teaching methods.
4. Assessing electronic resources.

HEALTH EDUCATOR

Faith Community Nursing: Scope and Standards of Practice (American Nurses Association & Health Ministries

Association, 2005) addresses health education in Standard of Practice 5B: Health Teaching and Health Promotion: "The faith community nurse employs strategies to promote health, wellness, and a safe environment" (p. 15). The Measurement Criteria for Standard 5B for FCN's are:

- Provides health teaching that addresses such topics as spiritual practices for health and healing, healthy lifestyles, risk reducing behaviors, developmental needs, activities of daily living, and preventive self-care.
- Uses health promotion and health teaching methods appropriate to the situation, the faith community, and the patient's spiritual beliefs and practices, developmental level, learning needs, readiness, and ability to learn language or communication preference or culture.
- Supports beliefs and practices of the faith community when selecting information and programs.
- Evaluates health information resources for use with faith community nursing for accuracy, readability, comprehensibility by patients, and congruence with patient's spiritual beliefs and practices.
- Seeks ongoing opportunities for feedback and evaluation of the effectiveness of health education and health promotion strategies.

FCNs may choose to conduct health education classes personally, or they may arrange for other professionals to conduct them. Available resources, the nature of the content, and time constraints will affect these decisions.

Theoretical content about teaching and learning has varied greatly across undergraduate and graduate nursing curricula. This chapter provides how-to information about teaching and learning to novice educators. Readers with teaching expertise should skim this chapter for new resources.

Federal initiatives have existed since the 1960s for health promotion and disease prevention. *Healthy People 1990, 2000, 2010,* and now *2020* sets objectives for the nation's health.

========================*FAST FACTS in a NUTSHELL*

The overarching goals of *Healthy People* are to:

• Achieve high quality, longer lives free of preventable disease, disability, injury, and premature death.
• Achieve health equity, eliminate disparities, and improve the health of all groups.
• Create social and physical environments that promote good health for all.
• Promote quality of life, healthy development, and healthy behaviors across all life stages.

In the past 20 years, there have been positive changes in the health of Americans. Mortality as a result of heart disease, stroke, cancer, and HIV has continued to decline, cholesterol levels have dropped, and tobacco use has declined. On the negative side, obesity is prevalent at all ages, diabetes incidence has increased, the teen birth rate has increased, and 33% of children under 3 years of age have not received basic vaccinations (*Health,* United States, 2010).

HEALTH AND BEHAVIOR CHANGE

========================*FAST FACTS in a NUTSHELL*

Important Definitions

• *Health promotion:* Behavior motivated by a desire to increase one's well-being and actualize wholeness, or *shalom.*
• *Health education:* Planned learning experiences that enable individuals, families, and communities to acquire information and skills with which to make informed health choices and decisions.
• *Faith-based health education:* Health education delivered in the context of the worldview of the faith tradition, incorporating prayer, Scripture, and worship.

Glanz, Rimer, and Viswanath (2008) state that health education includes instructional activities and strategies to change behavior, as well as organizational efforts, policies, resources, media, and community programs. The goal of health education is to provide clients with theory-based information from which to make informed health decisions and lifestyle choices. Positive health promotion choices prevent acute and chronic diseases, decrease disability, and enhance wellness. Glanz et al. posit that two ideas are critical to health education. The first is that behavior is affected by multiple levels of influence, which include individual, interpersonal, organizational community, and public policy factors. The second is that reciprocal causation occurs between individuals and environments. Behavior *influences* and *is influenced* by the social environment. The idea of reciprocal causation can help explain the positive correlation found between religion and health.

The field of health education recognizes many theoretical approaches to and models of health related behaviors. Glanz et al. suggest that different theoretical approaches are suited to different contexts.

Constructs that cut across the theories of health education Glanz et al.:

- The importance of the individual's worldview
- Multiple levels of influence on behavior
- Behavioral change as a process
- Motivation versus intention
- Intention versus action
- Changing behavior and maintaining change

The faith-based approach is a critical worldview element to faith community nursing. It provides both the rationale and the incentive for health promotion and disease activities related to the stewardship of the body.

THEORETICAL MODELS OF HEALTH BEHAVIOR

The Health Belief Model

The Health Belief Model (HBM) has been the most popu-
lar model for the past 5 decades. It was developed in the
1950s by a group of social psychologists working for the U.S.
Public Health Service who were trying to explain why people were not using free services available for TB screening.
Later, the model was extended to include people's reactions
to symptoms and compliance (or not) with prescribed medical regimes. Glanz et al. (2008) classify the HBM as a *value-
expectancy theory*.

According to the HBM, a person has a desire to avoid
illness or to recover from illness. This is perceived as the
value. The *expectation* is a belief that a specific health
action available to the person would or could prevent or
lessen illness. The expectation also includes a person's
estimate of personal susceptibility to a condition and the
potential severity of the condition. It is generally thought
that people will take positive action to prevent, screen
for, or control health conditions if they believe that they
are susceptible, that the illness could have serious consequences, that a course of action available would be of
benefit to lessen their susceptibility or the severity of the
disease, and that the barriers and costs of taking action are
outweighed by the benefits (p. 47). Many research studies,
both retrospective and prospective, show that perceived
barriers are the most powerful HBM aspects in explaining
or predicting health protective behaviors. Perceived susceptibility has also been shown to be an important pre-
dictor of preventive behaviors.

Pender's Health Promotion Model

Pender's Health Promotion Model (HPM) first appeared in
the nursing literature in the early 1980s. It was originally

proposed as a framework for integrating nursing and the behavioral sciences' perspectives on health behaviors. The HPM has been refined over time and is defined as a competence or approach-oriented model. Unlike the HBM, it does not address fear and threat as sources of motivation for healthful behavior. Because fear and threat are of limited value when working with children and teens, the HPM can be used across the lifespan (Pender, Murdaugh, & Parsons, 2011). The HPM integrates several constructs from the expectancy-value theory of motivation with social cognitive theory within a nursing perspective of holistic human functioning. The variables of this models include:

- *Individual Perceptions:*
  - Perceived susceptibility to a particular disease or perceived severity of a disease
- *Modifying Factors:*
  - Demographic variables (age, sex, race, ethnicity etc.)
  - Sociopsychological variables (personality, social class, peer and reference groups)
  - Structural variables (knowledge about the disease, prior experience with the disease)
  - Perceived threat of a particular disease
  - Cues to action such as media campaigns, reminder cards, illnesses of family members or friends
- *Likelihood of Action:*
  - Perceived benefits of preventive action–Perceived barriers to preventive action = Likelihood of taking action

Theories of health behavior are important to FCNs because they provide guidance in planning activities that will influence positive health behaviors and lifestyle changes. FCNs can use either of these models in planning. Several other health behavior models are available in the literature, but space prevents a detailed discussion.

NURSING INTERVENTIONS FOR HEALTH BEHAVIOR CHANGE

Pender et al. (2011) have identified nursing strategies for health behavioral change. These strategies include:

- *Raising consciousness*: By seeking and gaining information, observing others, and interpreting information in view of one's own circumstances, positive behavioral changes can occur.
- *Reevaluation of self*: This creates an awareness of discrepancies between one's values and beliefs and behaviors. Adherence to self-standards increases self-concept through feelings of pride and satisfaction. FCNs can help clients with self-reevaluation by suggesting possible activities or goals after making a healthy behavior change. Prayer and spiritual care can easily be incorporated into this strategy.
- *Promoting self-efficacy*: This refers to beliefs in personal capabilities to carry out a given behavior. The FCN can facilitate the client's successful performance of a behavior and give positive reinforcement, as well as help the client in identifying barriers to successful performance of a task and model the target behavior.
- *Enhancing the benefits of change*: Providing positive feedback encourages the repetition of desired behaviors and provides motivation for behavioral change.
- *Positive feedback:* This can be tangible, social, self-generated, or spiritual. Immediate and continuous positive reinforcement is highly desirable in the early phases of behavioral change. Intermittent reinforcement applied later stabilizes the behavior and makes it more resistant to extinction.
- *Controlling the environment:* Modifying the environment to stimulate and support healthful behavioral change provides cues that will trigger certain behaviors. Learning what environmental cues trigger positive or negative behaviors informs planning and interventions.

- *Dealing with barriers to change:* The FCN can help clients minimize real and perceived barriers to healthful behaviors by assessing the situation, clarifying information, correcting misinformation, and providing support services.
- *Maintaining the new behavior:* The FCN can help the client to maintain the new behavior in the setting in which it was learned and to generalize the behavior to other settings.

THE HEALTH EDUCATION PROCESS

Assessing the Learning Needs of the Congregation

Assessing learners is the first step of planning health education programs for faith communities.

================*FAST FACTS in a NUTSHELL*

A congregational assessment tool provides the FCN with quantitative data about:

- Incidence and types of chronic diseases that exist in the faith community
- Demographics of the faith community (ages, education levels)
- Formal committee structures within the faith community
- Interests of the membership about health topics
- Scheduling preferences of the membership for health programming

Kreps, Barnes, and Thackeray (2009) suggest that *audience analysis* includes people's needs, wants, motivational and resistance points, general attitudes, behaviors, and preferences related to health problems. It includes what they know, what they fear, and how they will likely react to specific learning methods. FCNs design health education programs using the congregational data analysis to develop programs that will meet the needs of the congregation. Kreps et al. define *channel analysis* as the process that helps determine which communication methods will most likely appeal to a target audience. This includes the setting where the audience is most easily reached, the method(s) in which they receive most of their information, and their preferences for communication methods.

A learning need is a gap between what someone currently knows and what he or she needs to know because of a lack of knowledge, skill, or attitude.

Age Considerations

The FCN needs to plan programs with consideration for the key elements of age, literacy level, and culture. Teaching principles differ for children and for adults. It is helpful for the FCN to review these principles as part of program planning.

Preschool Age Learners

Morrison (2009) suggests the following principles for teaching health promotion to preschool children:

- Children learn best when they use all their senses.
- Teachers should show love and respect for all children.
- Good teaching is based on theory, philosophy, goals, and objectives.
- Children's learning is enhanced by the use of concrete materials.
- Teaching should be child-centered.
- Teaching should move from the concrete to the abstract.
- Teaching should be based on the children's interests.
- Keep teaching sessions short, no longer than 15 minutes.

- Use storytelling as a teaching method.
- Give children tangible rewards to reinforce learning.

School-Age Children and Teenage Learners

Bastable and Dart (2008) recommend the following strategies for teaching school-age children and teenagers:

- Use diagrams and models, pictures, videos, and printed materials.
- Use materials that portray peers.
- Clarify terminology.
- Use analogies.
- Encourage participation.
- Provide reinforcement.
- Share decision making when appropriate.
- Suggest options.
- Be flexible.

Adults

Adult education is a collegial relationship between teacher and student rather than an expert-to-novice relationship. The emphasis for adult learning is related to life tasks and social roles. For learning to be relevant, adults need to see the benefits to be gained through the enterprise of learning. Adults are self-directed learners who bring a wealth of previous experience and knowledge to the learning experience.

Knowles, Holton, and Swanson (1998) provide the following principles for teaching adult learners. Adults:

- Need know why they need to learn something before undertaking it.
- Are self-directed.
- Have various life experiences that need to be incorporated into learning experiences.
- Have a life-centered or problem-centered orientation to learning.

- Have intrinsic motivators to learn, such as a sense of satisfaction.

======================================*FAST FACTS in a NUTSHELL*

Assessing learning needs includes the following steps:
- Identify the learner.
- Choose the right setting to collect the data.
- Collect the data from the targeted audience.
- Prioritize needs for knowledge as mandatory, desirable, or possible.
- Determine the availability of educational resources and the number of materials needed.

11

Teaching in Faith Community Nursing Practice

INTRODUCTION

FCNs need to carefully assess literacy levels of printed health education materials and prepare their own user-friendly instructional materials based on the literacy levels and ages of those they instruct. FCNs also should carefully plan where, when, and how best to conduct instructional programs for members of the faith community to achieve positive outcomes.

In this chapter, you will learn:

1. How to assess the literacy levels of written instructional materials.
2. Where and when to plan educational programs.
3. How to develop and use a variety of instructional materials.

LITERACY LEVELS

Literacy is a broad term used to describe socially required and expected reading and writing skills, including the ability to understand printed or written materials commonly encountered in daily life. Doak, Doak, and Root (1996) state that the commonly accepted definition of *literacy* is the ability to read, understand, and interpret information written at the 8th-grade level. They define *low literacy* as adults' ability to read, write, and comprehend information between 5th and 8th grade levels and *functional illiteracy* as having reading, writing, and comprehension skills below the 5th-grade level.

═══════════════════════════════*FAST FACTS in a NUTSHELL*

Fisher (1999) categorizes literacy into three general tasks:

- *Prose tasks:* Measure reading comprehension and the ability to extract themes from newspapers, magazines, poems, and books.
- *Document tasks:* Assess the ability to interpret documents, such as insurance reports, consent forms, and transportation schedules.
- *Quantitative tasks:* Assess the ability to work with numerical information embedded in written materials, such as computing restaurant bills, interpreting paycheck information, and counting calories.

The American Medical Association (AMA), Institute of Medicine (IOM), and Healthy People 2010 have adopted the following definition of health literacy: "The degree to which individuals have the capacity to obtain, process and understand basic health information and services needed to make appropriate health decisions" (Ratzan & Parker, 2000). The AMA added to this definition by concluding the sentence with "and follow instructions for treatment." The AMA Website has an entire section on health literacy and its implications for health and compliance with medical regimes. Toolkits and continuing education programs are available for clinicians.

ASSESSING READABILITY OF HEALTH EDUCATION MATERIALS

FCNs should carefully assess literacy levels of printed health education materials. Doak et al. (1996) recommend that instructional materials be written at the 5th-grade level. Bastable (2008) notes that over 40 formulas can measure readability of printed materials.

The Spache Grade Level Score (Spache, 1953) focuses on evaluating material for children at grade levels 1–3. The SMOG formula is a valid, simple, and fast method for assessing readability of material from grade 4 through college level. This method is based on 100% reading comprehension, meaning that if the SMOG formula assesses reading material at the 8th-grade level, all readers at the 8th-grade level could comprehend the material.

Most word processing software can assess the readability of a document. Microsoft Word 2010 uses the Flesch Reading Ease Test and the Flesch-Kincaid Grade Level Test. Both are options in the Spell Check tool. The Reading Ease Test rates text on a 100-point scale. The higher the score, the easier it is to understand the document. The Flesch-Kincaid Grade Level Test rates text on U.S. schools' grade levels. For example, a score of 8.0 means that 8th-graders can understand the document.

PREPARING USER-FRIENDLY PRINTED HEALTH EDUCATION MATERIALS

Using the following points as a guide will assist you in preparing clear and effective health education materials:

- Put the most important information first and make it boldface or italics.
- Use a simple, easy-to-read font.
- Keep sentences short.
- Write in an active voice using the present tense.
- Write in a conversational style; use personal pronouns *you* and *your*.

- Focus on only one concept per paragraph.
- Leave plenty of white space between paragraphs.
- Define terms clearly and use them consistently.
- Convert medical terminology to lay terms.
- Use numbers and statistics sparingly.

WHEN, WHERE, AND HOW TO TEACH

The "when" of providing a health education program depends on data collected from the faith community regarding preferences for days and times. The FCN should be aware of local events and peak vacation weeks that might conflict with program scheduling as well. The "where" for health programs depends on the availability of appropriate space in the physical facilities of the congregation. Ideally, rooms should comfortably accommodate the expected size of the audience. If there will be small group discussions, separate spaces need to be available. Depending on the faith community's structure, the rooms may need to be reserved in advance of use. The setting up and breaking down of rooms must be planned for, and volunteer assistance may need to be recruited.

Ideally, spaces for educational programs should be well ventilated, temperature controlled, and equipped with the appropriate audiovisual media equipment. Spaces need adequate lighting and sound system, and be accessible to persons with disabilities. If health screening activities are part of a planned program, privacy for actual screening procedures is required. Portable screens can be used if separate rooms are not available.

═══════════════════════════*FAST FACTS in a NUTSHELL*

Using Hansen and Fisher's (1998) acronym TEACH as a guide to ensure that health teaching is effective:

T = Tune in to the learner's thoughts and needs, and address the learner's priorities for learning first.

Continued

Continued

E = Edit information to focus on "must know" content.

A = Act on teachable moments. Teach at every opportunity.

C = Clarify often and verify your assumptions by seeking frequent feedback from the learner.

H = Honor the learner as a partner. Build learning on the learner's prior experiences and share responsibility for the educational process.

Instructional methods are the "how" of teaching. Decisions about instructional methods should be made based on variables such as how active or passive the learner will be and how much control the teacher wants to have during the learning experience.

When considering the instructional method to use in your health care teaching, keep in mind the following hierarchy of learner retention reported by Cohen (1991). : Learners retain:

- 5% from lecture
- 10% from reading
- 20% from audiovisual materials
- 30% from discussion
- 50% from demonstration
- 75% from practice by doing
- 90% by teaching others

Based on this information, FCNs should focus on learning activities that use a mixture of instructional styles with as much active learning as possible.

≡ *FAST FACTS in a NUTSHELL*

Instructional Methods

Lectures	Games
Discussions	Simulation
One-on-one instruction	Role-playing
Demonstrations/return	Role-modeling
self-instruction	Computer-assisted
	instruction

Lectures

Lectures are considered the most economical and efficient instructional method because a large number of people get the same information at the same time. This method is unidirectional, going from teacher to learners, and learners have passive roles.

Lectures are organized with an introduction, body, and summary or conclusion. The introduction should engage learners with the topic to be addressed and build rapport between the speaker and audience. The body of a lecture contains the content of the presentation and is delivered using a prepared outline. Examples the audience can relate to are included in the body, helping the audience link new information with information that is familiar to them. Lectures are often complemented with PowerPoint slides.

Tips for Preparing PowerPoint Slides

- Limit each slide to one concept.
- Use the 6 x 6 rule: 6 or fewer lines per slide and 6 or fewer words per line.
- Use single words and short phrases.
- Slide headings, font size, and styles should be consistent throughout.
- Title fonts should be large: 38–40 points.
- Text fonts should be a minimum of 24 points.
- PowerPoint provides coordinating font colors: use them!

- Show no more than 2 slides per minute.
- Create a notes page so you do not have to turn your back on the audience.
- Use animation sparingly, if at all. It becomes annoying to the viewer quickly!
- Avoid clip art. Use free photographs from Websites.

Keep the purpose of the presentation and expected learning outcomes in mind when developing the body of a presentation. Be careful to avoid information overload! Keep the presentation simple, and repeat key points with examples. In the conclusion or summary, review and highlight key points that the audience will take home. If there is a question-and-answer period at the end, repeat questions asked, so that all can hear.

Group Discussions

Group discussions, by definition, are an instructional method whereby learners get together to exchange information, opinions, and/or feelings with each other and the teacher. It is among the most frequently used instructional methods and is economical and efficient. Fitzgerald (2008) considers group discussion an effective method for learning in both the cognitive and affective domains. Groups can be small or large, depending on the purpose. Tang, Funnell, and Anderson (2006) suggest a group size of 10 as ideal.

To direct a discussion, give the group clear learning objectives and questions for discussion. The teacher's role is to facilitate the discussion and to summarize and highlight key points, as well as to model respectful attention in participating in the group.

Individual Instruction

One-on-one instruction is time consuming but, as Fitzgerald (2008) states, it allows for questioning, an excellent method

to use for teaching, as it makes the single learner participate actively and the teacher can give immediate feedback.
FCNs may find themselves in many situations where they
will engage in one-on-one instruction.

Games

Games are an instructional method whereby learners participate in competitive activities with rules. Games can be simple or complex. The teacher acts as facilitator, awards prizes
to the winners, and debriefs the group, stressing the lessons
of the experience and helping the group evaluate the game
experience. Games can be purchased or designed specifically for learning. Well-known games such as *Jeopardy* and
Trivial Pursuit can be modified to meet learning objectives.

When planning to use games, be sure to consider group
size, time constraints, and both the educational and literacy
levels of the learners. Prior to using a game in a real situation, pilot test it with a small group. This will help you to
identify any issues or difficulties in following the rules, as
well as how long it takes to complete the game.

ELECTRONIC RESOURCES

Every day, more and more people use the Internet to access
health information. Web-based information can be retrieved
easily and quickly in the privacy of one's home or office.
Web access has caused both an information explosion and
information overload. FCNs can help members of the faith
community assess and evaluate the integrity of Web-based
resources by using and understanding the Health on the Net
Foundations Principles (www.healthonthenet.org). These
principles include evaulating:

- *Authority:* Health care advice should be given by professionals. The Website should provide the qualifications
  of authors.

- *Complementarity:* The information provided should support, not replace, the relationship between patients and their health care providers.
- *Confidentiality:* There should be respect for the privacy of site users.
- *Attribution:* Information provides clear citations to source data and dates. The date when the Webpage was last modified is clear.
- *Justifiability:* Any claims to benefits or performance of a specific treatment, commercial product, or service are supported by appropriate, balanced evidence.
- *Transparency:* The information is accessible with valid contact details.
- *Financial disclosure:* The Website should provide details of its funding.
- *Advertising:* Advertisements are clearly distinguishable from editorial content.

═══════════════════════════*FAST FACTS in a NUTSHELL*

The Health on the Web Code (HONcode) is used by over 7,300 certified Websites, more than 10 million pages in 102 countries. It is internationally known for its pioneering work in the field of health information ethics (www.healthonthenet.org).

12

Program Planning

INTRODUCTION

As discussed in Chapter 9, assessment of the faith community provides data from which to plan health promotion and disease prevention programs. The assessment data informs the FCN of the interest areas and needs of the faith community. A good beginning is to look at the list of interest areas and needs and prioritize which programs can achieve early success. Things to consider are the size of the issue (number of people affected), the ease or difficulty of meeting the need or addressing the issue, and resources available to the FCN.

In this chapter you will learn:

1. How to plan a health program in a faith community.
2. How to implement health program in a faith community.
3. How to evaluate a health program in a health community.

TYPES OF PROGRAMS

The types and scope of health education programs depend upon the resources of the faith community. Types of programs include health screening, health monitoring, health education, health fairs, guest speakers, and support groups. Congregations with well-established health ministries and volunteer structures will be able to provide a broader range of offerings than a small congregation with a part-time volunteer parish nurse.

Blood pressure screening and monitoring programs are often provided to faith communities by their nurses. This is an activity that can take place right after a worship service. It requires a minimum of equipment and can be done quickly. A follow-up system is critical for members with elevated readings. This activity, which can be carried out by one or more nurses, is interactive and nonthreatening, and helps the FCN and congregants to become familiar with one another. Figure 12.1 provides the steps for setting up a blood pressure screening and monitoring program.

========================*FAST FACTS in a NUTSHELL*

If pocket cards for BP recordings are not available they can be made. For example:

Applewood Community Church Member: _____

Blood Pressure Monitoring Program

Date	B/P		Date	B/P
____	____		____	____
____	____		____	____

Faith community assessment data provide direction for planning the content of health promotion and disease prevention programs. Programs can be advertised in the church bulletin, the faith community Website, and in community newsletters. Flyers can be posted on bulletin boards. Encouraging the pastor to mention upcoming events always has a positive effect on participation! In addition, the FCN can create a resource center of health-related print materials and/or lists of Websites. The FCN should assess the

Figure 12.1   How to Start a Blood Pressure
Screening and Monitoring Program

- Review the faith community assessment data to determine risk for hypertension and the numbers of members who identify themselves as hypertensive.
- Determine the availability of voluntary help from other nurses in the faith community to assist in taking and recording results.
- Determine the availability of lay volunteers willing to assist in record keeping.
- Once the frequency and time (ideally, after a worship service) are established, arrange for a relatively quiet but convenient setting to conduct the program.
- Obtain needed equipment (BP cuffs, stethoscopes, records notebook or laptop).
- Obtain brochures about hypertension and pocket cards for BP recordings from the local chapter of the American Heart Association.
- Publicize the event with signs and in the worship service bulletin.
- At the event, have volunteers help with recording and distributing literature.
- Encourage participants to attend the next screening.
- After the event, meet with the health ministry team to evaluate the event.

literacy level and cultural sensitivity of all print materials and Websites.

Another way to structure health programs for a faith community is to use the federal health observances calendar, available at www.healthfinder.gov. Appendix A illustrates how this might be used as a program planning guide. The Website also provides a monthly toolkit that includes sample announcements, sample tweets, e-cards, Web badges, and resources. Local chapters of national organizations such as the American Heart Association and the American Automobile Association can provide resources for program development and program materials. Other local resources include the police, fire, and health departments, which provide prevention programs (fire, crime), how-to programs (such as infant-seat installation), and health education services.

GUEST SPEAKERS

Volunteer or paid guest speakers may be invited to provide information for health programs of faith communities. Guest speakers should be experts on the topic to be presented, and every effort should be made to make the event as user friendly to the guest speaker as possible. The FCN is responsible for making sure that the event is well publicized and that there is an audience for the presentation. Figure 12.2 provides a timeline for planning a health education event with a guest speaker.

When the FCN is aware of interest in a particular topic, such as exercise or stress management, weight management, or healthful meals, the development of support groups or specific activity groups may be beneficial to the interested members. While the FCN would provide resources and guidance to these types of groups, it is not reasonable or possible to expect the FCN to attend every session. Durrant and Rieckmann (2009) believe that the strength of using support groups as intervention is helping a person gain objective insight into personal behavior as well as realize that one is not alone in trying to cope with a particular problem. Insight comes with the group's feedback, and group membership provides a sense of community. The element of *faith* also gives an array of resources for support groups, including but not limited to prayer and reflection.

Figure 12.2   Steps for Planning a Health Education
Event with a Guest Speaker

3 Months Prior to the Event
- Determine the objectives of the event.
- Consider the expected size of the audience.
- Consider potential dates and times for the event and check availability of rooms.
- Contact the guest speaker, confirm a date and time for the event, ask about any requirements for audiovisual hardware, and clarify who will provide it.
- Reserve the appropriately sized room and arrange for hardware if needed.

1 Month Prior to the Event
- Reconfirm date and time with the guest speaker. Obtain handouts to be copied.
- Publicize the event with inserts in worship bulletins, flyers on bulletin boards, and the faith community Website.
- Ask the faith community leader to endorse the event.
- Register participants.
- Create a program evaluation form.
- Solicit volunteer help, if needed.

1 Week Before the Event
- Reconfirm date and time with the guest speaker.
- Review room setup plans.
- Make any needed signs.
- Duplicate handouts as needed.

Continued

Figure 12.2 *Continued*

Day of the Event
- Place any needed signs.
- Test audiovisual equipment
- Meet and greet guest speakers and participants.
- Provide and collect evaluation forms.

After the Event
- Review program evaluation forms.
- Send thank-you notes to the guest speaker and volunteers who helped.

HEALTH FAIRS

Health fairs are events that bring people and health professionals together to provide health education, screening, counseling and referral, and follow-up. Health fairs can target specific age groups or not. They can be large events with many participants and activities or small events focused on a specific issue or disease. A faith community's size may affect whether a health fair is open to the public or only to the faith community. Small congregations may coordinate a health fair with another faith community.

═══════════════════════════*FAST FACTS in a NUTSHELL*

Health fairs are events that generally provide:

- Increased health awareness by providing screenings, activities, materials, demonstrations, and information.
- More awareness of local, state, and federal health services and resources.

Continued

Continued

- Motivation to the participants to make positive health behavior changes.
- Instruction on self-care practices.
- Identification of interest areas for future programs.

Patterson (2003) states that health fairs make a health ministry accessible and visible. She reports that a health fair is one the first events that clergy and health cabinets want to see take place with a new faith community nursing program. Boyes (2001) suggests that health fairs encourage wellness in a festive atmosphere. Exhibits, demonstrations, classes, screenings, activities, speakers, puppet shows, food samples, and speakers provide information to help congregants make healthful choices. Boyes describes a health fair she developed with the theme "wholeness"—quite apt for the mission of health ministry. Figure 12.3 provides steps to plan a health fair.

Figure 12.3   How to Plan a Health Fair

6 to 12 Months Prior to the Event
- Choose the event theme (broad, such as fitness, or narrow, such as heart health).
- Develop goals and objectives.
- Choose a date and time for the event.
- Select a chairman and establish a planning committee.
- Choose and reserve an appropriate site. Consider availability of parking and access for persons with disabilities.

Continued

Figure 12.3 *Continued*

- Assign tasks among committee members. Typical tasks include clinical participants, food procurement, volunteers, door prizes, publicity, promotional items or giveaways, facilities, and equipment.
- Select screenings and services to be offered.
- Review liability insurance and HIPPA needs.

3 to 6 Months Prior to the Event
- Establish timelines.
- Secure commitments from health care providers and exhibitors.
- Secure volunteers, including greeters, registration table staff, and photographer.
- Reserve any rental equipment needed.
- Make a referral plan for screening findings needing immediate attention.

3 Months Prior to the Event
- Order educational materials as needed.
- Purchase or solicit donation of prizes, decoration, giveaways, and tablecloths.
- Reserve trash receptacles.
- Make poster and flyers.
- Copy print material (registration/evaluations forms, blood pressure record cards).
- Provide written confirmation to all participants, including day and time for setup, a map and directions to the setting, and general guidelines for the event.
- Publicize "Save the date."

1 Month Prior to the Event
- Meet with the planning committee to review implementation plans.

Continued

Figure 12.3 *Continued*

- Publicize the event within the faith community and externally if open to public.
- Secure supplies such as extension cords, pens, markers, paper products, and tape.
- Map out a floor plan of booths and activity areas.
- Make signs.
- Make a program, acknowledging exhibitors, volunteers, donors, etc.

1 Day Prior to the Event
- Set up tables, booths, and chairs.
- Set up the registration table.
- Set up the food area.
- Set up equipment as needed.

Day of the Event
- Direct and instruct volunteers
- Collect registration and evaluation forms.
- Check in participants.
- Say a prayer.

After the Event
- Send thank-you notes to volunteers, donors, and professional participants.
- Tabulate evaluation data.
- Report back to the health ministry team.

Wurzbach (2004) describes a model health fair as having four elements:

- *Health education:* Should be delivered in interactive ways.
- *Screening:* The longest lines at health fairs are for blood pressure, height/weight/BMI, anemia tests, and visual acuity tests.

- *Counseling and referral:* Allow a professional to out-line actions needed to improve wellness and encourage healthful lifestyle changes.
- *Follow-up:* Can be done by mailings or phone, with prior permission.

Durban (2003) cautions that a new FCN should not attempt a heath fair in the first year of service, unless much assistance is readily available. Ideally, the health ministry team is involved in event planning. The FCN should be responsible for choosing the focus or theme of the health fair and for compiling a list of potential participating agencies and organizations. Wilson (2000) advises that at least three nurses be available at blood pressure screening areas to avoid lines and suggests that church members serve as greeters and guides. Because health fairs require so much planning and time, it is essential that adequate time and volunteers are available throughout the process. Figure 12.4 provides a checklist for a successful health fair.

Figure 12.4   Checklist for a Successful Health Fair

- *Site:* Consider access roads, restroom facilities, parking, lighting, electrical outlet availability, and access for persons with disabilities.
- *Layout:* If possible, plan for a single entry point at which participants register. Allow for private space and extra space around screening areas for lines to form.
- *Materials:* List all needed equipment/supplies (first-aid, restroom paper products.
- *Registration:* Greeters usher people to the registration table. Forms include any needed consents (follow-up), HIPPA Notice of Privacy Practices, and evaluations.

Continued

Figure 12.4 *Continued*

- *Photos:* Someone can take photos, which can be used to publicize the next event.
- *Timing:* Check both the faith community and local community calendars before scheduling the event to prevent a conflict that might affect attendance.
- *Exhibitors:* Confirm all participants, their space and equipment needs, and arrival time needed for setup by phone or e-mail the week before the event.
- *Giveaways:* Plastic bags make it easy for participants to collect printed materials. Other giveaways should support the theme of the event.
- *Directions:* Post direction signs to parking, entry, exits, restrooms, registration.
- *Cleanup:* A committee and scheduled timeframe for cleanup activities are needed.
- *Thanks:* Thank all involved formally in writing. Send exhibitors evaluation forms.
- *Evaluation:* Registration document attendance. Providers report the number of people screened and referred for follow-up. Analyze evaluation data and use to plan the next event.

===================*FAST FACTS in a NUTSHELL*

Web Resources for Planning Health Fairs

- http://fcs.tamu.edu/health/health_fair_planning_guide/activity_ideas.php
- http://www.cdc.gov/women/planning/fair.htm

Continued

Continued

- http://www.wellnessproposals.com/health_fair_
  wellness_fair_planning_guide/activities_and_ideas.
  htm
- http://www.aarc.org/headlines/10/04/year_of_the_
  lung/health_fair.pdf
- http://www.capta.org/sections/programs/
  downloads/h-events.pdf

Meeting Diverse
Community Needs

13

Meeting Special Needs in the Faith Community

INTRODUCTION

FCNs are called upon to provide spiritual care as well as traditional nursing care, both in institutional settings and in the home, to congregants who suffer from chronic illness, have had surgery, or have had an accident. After conducting a holistic assessment of a patient who is chronically ill, a FNC can help the patient and his or her family cope with the disease and can provide comfort by listening, just being present, reading Scripture, and/or praying.

In this chapter you will learn:

1. How to provide spiritual care to those who have acute illness, have undergone surgery, or have been in an accident.
2. How to conduct holistic assessments of patients with chronic disease and provide care for them and their families.
3. How to satisfy the spiritual needs of patients with chronic illness.

ACUTE CARE, SURGERIES, AND ACCIDENTS

Depending on the structure of the health ministry, the FCN may be called upon to visit congregants and their families in their homes, as well as in a variety of institutional settings, as they deal with acute illnesses, surgeries, or the outcomes of accidents. These situations require the FCN to assume the roles of integrator of faith and health, health educator, personal health counselor, health advocate, and referral agent.

As a congregant and his or her family are dealing with a crisis or—at minimum—a transitional situation, the FCN must be cognizant of crisis intervention skills, as well as spiritual assessment and the provision of spiritual care. The spiritual needs of adults suffering from acute illness vary, depending on factors such as age, religious tradition, and severity of the illness. The FCN must do a spiritual assessment and assist in meeting the presenting spiritual needs of patient and family. Sternberg (2009) suggests that hospitals can actually become "healing spaces" if appropriate attention is paid to the spiritual needs of patients and families.

═══════════════════════*FAST FACTS in a NUTSHELL*

Spiritual Care Resources for FCNs

Darby, M. (2004). *Reflections on the hands of a nurse: A book of prayers and reflections for nurses.* Omaha, NE: Surprise Publishing.

Driscol, M. (2006). *Devotions for caregivers: A month's supply of prayer.* Mahwah, NJ: Paulist Press.

Feist-Heilmeier, C. (2008). *Nurse are from heaven: Nurses through the eyes of faith.* Longwood, FL: Xulon Press.

Morris, G. S. (2004). *I am the Lord who heals you.* Nashville, TN: Abington Press.

Continued

Continued

O'Brien, M. E. (2003). *Prayer in nursing: The spirituality of compassionate caregiving.* Sudbury, MA: Jones & Bartlett.

O'Brien, M. E. (2008). *A sacred covenant: The spiritual ministry of nursing.* Sudbury, MA: Jones & Bartlett.

Patterson, D. (2005). *Healing words for healing people.* Cleveland: Pilgrim Press.

Patterson, D. (2009). *The healing word: Preaching and Teaching Health Ministry.* Cleveland: Pilgrim Press.

Schuler, L. L. (2006). *Visitation handbook for christian parish nurses.* Victoria, BC, Canada: Trafford Publishing.

Shelly, J. A. (1979). *Caring in crisis: Bible studies for helping people.* Downers Grove, IL: InterVarsity Press.

Sudden, unanticipated acute illness may pose serious emotional and spiritual problems related to fear of possible death or disability. Psychological depression may result from severe pain or fatigue. A patient may question God's will and/or express anger at God for allowing the illness to happen. The FCN can help others in the instituitional setting be attuned to the patient's spiritual needs and provide spiritual care to the patient as well. Listening, being present, reading Scripture or praying may comfort the patient.

Carson (2008) proposes three broad categories of ministries to provide spiritual care. She defines *ministry* as "the use of our gifts, talents, time, and energy in the service to another" (p. 137). These ministries are:

- *Ministry of presence*: Involves a willingness to be an active listener—empathetic, vulnerable, humble, and committed.
- *Ministry of the word*: Involves a willingness to conduct a spiritual assessment, to discuss religious concerns, to

offer verbal support and encouragement, and to make a referral to the chaplain or preferred faith community leader, to use prayer and scripture as a means of alleviating spiritual distress, and to advocate for the patient's spiritual beliefs in the health care setting.
• *Ministry of action*: Involves a willingness to take action on behalf of a patient's spiritual needs (pp. 138–139).

CHRONIC DISEASE NEEDS

The U.S. Center for Health Statistics defines a chronic disease as lasting 3 months or more. Chronic diseases generally cannot be prevented by vaccines or cured by medication, nor do they just disappear. Health-damaging behaviors, particularly tobacco use, lack of physical activity, and poor eating habits, are major contributors to the leading chronic diseases, which tend to become more common with age. The leading chronic diseases in developed countries include (in alphabetical order) arthritis, cardiovascular disease such as heart attacks and stroke, cancer such as breast and colon cancer, diabetes, epilepsy and seizures, obesity, and oral health problems. These conditions plague older adults in the United States and other developed nations.

================*FAST FACTS in a NUTSHELL*

The Centers for Disease Control and Prevention (CDC, 2010) report that:

• One of two adults has at least one chronic disease, and 25% of these have limitations in one or more daily activities.
• Arthritis is the most common form of chronic disease, with 19 million people reporting activity limitations.

Continued

Continued

- Diabetes continues to be the leading cause of kidney failure, nontraumatic lower extremity amputation, and blindness among person aged 20–74.
- An estimated 75% of the nation's $2 trillion spent on medical costs was attributable to chronic disease in 2008.

Lubkin and Larsen (2005) remind us that the U.S. health care system is designed for acute and episodic care and generally provides this type of care efficiently and effectively. They identify *disease* as a condition that is viewed from a pathophysiological model, such as alterations in structure and function. *Illness* is defined as the human experience of symptoms and suffering, and it refers to how the disease is perceived, lived with, and responded to by individuals and their families. Understanding the illness experience is essential in providing holistic care (p. 4). Helping individuals and families cope with the illness experience is a key element of FCN practice.

==*FAST FACTS in a NUTSHELL*

Glaser and Strauss (1968) first introduced the term *trajectory* while studying dying patients in hospital settings. "A trajectory is defined as a course of illness over time, and the actions taken by clients, families, and health professionals to manage or shape that course" (Corbin, 2000, p. 3).

George (2006) believes that using an illness trajectory framework is helpful for caring for clients on a long-term basis because it allows the FCN to understand where the client is on the continuum of both disease and illness. Health care professionals tend to focus on symptoms and treatment, while the patient and family manage the illness experience. This experience includes controlling symptoms and performing the necessary everyday tasks to manage illness (Lubkin & Larsen 2005). George states that a FCN may serve as the interpreter between the professional, disease-oriented model and the individual and family coping with the illness experience.

While the CDC clearly stresses the importance of health promotion and disease prevention, a FCN spends a significant amount of time helping congregants manage their chronic diseases and live with their imitations. FCNs can institute a variety of screenings to identify conditions early and can provide health education programs about specific chronic diseases, such as "Tips for Living with Arthritis."

The Stanford University School of Medicine has developed a Chronic Disease Self-Management Program, which is a promising resource for FCNs. The program is 2.5 hours/week for 6 weeks. Each participant receives *Living a Healthy Life with Chronic Conditions* (3rd ed.) by Lorig, Holman, Sobel, Gonzalez, and Minor (2006), and the *Time for Healing* audiotape by Regan.

═══════════════════════*FAST FACTS in a NUTSHELL*

Stanford University's Chronic Disease Self-Management Program teaches:

- Techniques to deal with problems such as frustration, fatigue, pain, and isolation.
- Appropriate exercises to maintain and improve strength, flexibility, endurance.
- Appropriate use of medications.
- How to communicate effectively with family, friends, and health professionals.
- Nutrition.
- How to evaluate new treatments (http://patient eduction.stanford.edu).

A FCN uses faith community assessment data to understand the extent and types of chronic diseases present in the congregation. When working with patients and families coping with chronic disease, the FCN needs to conduct a holistic assessment of the patient, which will help the FCN identify and correct any knowledge deficits related to the disease. These may be addressed by the FCN, or the FCN may refer the family to educational programs in the community. The FCN may consider referring the patient and/or the family to support groups in the faith community or the larger community.

A FCN has opportunities to make home visits to congregants. Such visits help the FCN gain a holistic perspective of patients and families. Observing people in their home setting provides an accurate assessment of family processes, strengths, and weaknesses.

As community health nurses know, meeting a patient and family on their home "turf" changes the balance of power and provides the family with a sense of control. Pierce and Lutz (2005) report that autonomy and control are interrelated and that both are affected by the ability of professional providers to support family caregivers. Maintaining a chronically ill person in the home requires family caregiver responsibility.

The experience of a chronic illness may be a time when spiritual needs previously unnoticed or neglected become apparent (Baldacchino & Draper, 2001). Favor (2004) reports that spiritual beliefs and faith-based behavior play multiple roles in caregivers' lives. Spirituality involves not only connectedness with a sacred other, but also other people, perspectives, and sources of value and meaning beyond oneself. Stuckey (2001) reports that religious beliefs and practice are essential aspects of caregiving, and reliance on prayer is reported by many caregivers as a source of strength.

O'Brien (2011) states that personal spirituality or religious beliefs and practices may constitute an important mediating variable for the chronically ill. She proposes six spiritual needs in chronic illness (pp. 199–203):

- *Hope*: Hope is anticipation that something desired will occur. Shelly and Fish (1988) point out that placing one's hope in God does not mean an immediate end to suffering or anxiety, but rather trust in God's support during a crisis (p. 44).
- *Trust:* The idea of trust indicates confidence in something or someone. Johnson (1992) states that trusting for the ill person who is a believer will give a sense of security that God's healing power will be operative in his or her life (p. 92). O'Brien reminds us that the healing that occurs may be of a spiritual or emotional nature as opposed to physical healing.
- *Courage:* Emotional strength is not as the absence of fear, but rather "the ability to transcend one's fears, to choose to actively face what needs to be" (Stoll, 1989, p. 196).
- *Faith:* Faith means belief and trust in God.
- *Peace:* Peace is a sense of calm, a feeling of being undisturbed. It is a right relationship with God entailing forgiveness, reconciliation, and union (Dwyer, 1990).
- *Love:* Love is to care for or treasure; the unconditional love of God.

14

Loss and Grief

INTRODUCTION

The U.S. population is aging rapidly. In 2008, an estimated 39 million people were age 65 and older, accounting for just over 13% of the total population. By 2030, the size of this population is expected to be twice as large as in 2000, growing from 35 million to 72 million (Agingstats.gov). In 2007, this population accounted for 72.5% of all American deaths. Heart disease accounted for 28% of all deaths, followed by cancer (22%) and stroke (7%). Death from external causes (accidents, homicide, and suicide) were not in the top five causes of death for this age group. These data indicate that the vast majority of Americans die of natural causes in old age (CDC.gov).

In this chapter you will learn:

1. Legal documents and models that help a person plan for a dignified end of life.
2. Appropriate spiritual care for the end of life.
3. Issues to be considered in palliative and hospice care.
4. Planning and preparation for death at home.
5. Support for family and the faith community through the loss and grief process.

151

PLANNING FOR THE END OF LIFE

Rao, Anderson, and Smith (2002) believe that, as death now occurs at later ages and often as a result of protracted illness, quality at the end of life has become a societal concern and a public health issue. They describe the end of life as having three characteristics of other public health priorities: a high burden, a major impact, and the potential for preventing the suffering associated with illness.

Death With Dignity

When one thinks of the planning and health education that occurs during a pregnancy and the birthing process, comparatively little attention is paid to the dying process. Keegan and Drick (2011) believe that the greatest human freedom is to live and die according to one's wishes. Death with Dignity is a movement to provide options for the dying to control their own end-of-life care.

The states of Oregon and Washington have death with dignity acts that allow terminally ill adults to end their lives through voluntary self-administration of lethal medications, expressly prescribed by their physician for that purpose.

The Respectful Death Model is a research-based, holistic model developed from qualitative research findings of a study of cancer patients (Wasserman, 2008). This model recognizes the importance of relationships in end-of-life care, the stories of patients and families, and incorporating them into care planning. The stories are obtained within a therapeutic relationship using "mindful listening" (Farber & Farber, 2006, p. 223).

Lankarani-Fard et al. (2010) designed the Go Wish card game, which allows patients to consider the importance of common issues at the end of life. Of the 133 subjects, the value selected as most important was to be pain free. Other highly ranked values included spirituality, maintaining a sense of self, symptom management, and establishing strong relationships with health professionals. The average time for patients to rank the values was 22 minutes. These findings indicate that it is feasible to use this game to obtain a portrayal of a patient's care goals in a time-efficient manner.

FAST FACTS in a NUTSHELL

Keegan and Drick (2011) suggest the following advanced skills to foster meaningful conversation about the end of life:

- Speak from an open heart.
- Be in the moment.
- Acknowledge your feelings to yourself.
- Allow yourself to feel the feelings.
- Observe the inner shifting in your feelings as you listen and talk.

Keegan and Drick describe an alternative setting for the dying process called the Golden Room, a room designed with serenity and peace in its appointments and staffed by palliative care nurses who are well versed in integrative and holistic nursing practices. The setting and the nursing care honor the sacred rite of dying and support the person and his or her family on their journey from life to a peaceful death.

Advance Directives

Advance directives are legal documents that allow people to communicate in advance their desires for end-of-life care. Advanced directives detail the specific types of treatment that persons do or do not want (feeding tubes, CPR, etc.) if they cannot speak for themselves. Advance directives can be short, simple statements, either handwritten or completed on forms provided by health care agencies. They should be witnessed by a notary if possible. Most importantly, a family member and the attending physician should have copies. Advance directives can changed at any time, as long as the person is able to think rationally and communicate wishes clearly. State laws differ on advance directives, and it is always a good idea to have an attorney review the documents.

Living Wills

A living will is a type of advance directive. It is a written, legal document that describes the kind of medical or life-sustaining treatment(s) a person wants if he or she becomes seriously or terminally ill. A living will does not transfer decision-making authority to any other person.

With a living will, one can accept or refuse care that may include:

- The use of dialysis
- The use of ventilators
- Cardiac resuscitation
- Organ or tissue donation

Durable Power of Attorney

A durable power of attorney for health care is also an advance directive. It is a document that names another person as one' health care proxy. The proxy is given authority to make health decisions for a patient if the patient is unable to do so. It becomes active when a person is unconscious or unable to make medical decisions.

Do Not Resuscitate Order

A Do Not Resuscitate (DNR) order is another kind of advance directive. A DNR is a request not to have cardiopulmonary resuscitation (CPR) during cardiac arrest or if breathing stops. Without this documentation, hospitalized patients will be resuscitated.

SPIRITUAL CARE FOR THE END OF LIFE

The end-of-life literature is clear that the true presence, the being-there of family, nurses, physicians, and clergy is critically important to support a dying patient. Todd and Baldwin (2006), both palliative care nurses, believe the experience of dying has become institutionalized and that nurses should advocate for patients to take ownership of the dying process. They suggest that nurses encourage dying patients to accept the illness, reflect on the meaning of life, value close relationships, and mend what needs fixing.

FAST FACTS in a NUTSHELL

Todd and Baldwin encourage dying patients: "Paint a picture using the best-quality paints, show it your family, accept its difficulties, frame it in the context of your life, be proud of it, take ownership of it, and place it where it will remind your love ones of you." They call this the art of dying.

Dr. Aldebra Schroll (2010) writes in a personal reflection article that working in a hospice setting allows her to practice medicine holistically, with emphasis on the whole person from medical, spiritual, and social perspectives. It allows her to approach her patients in the context of family, with a collaborative team approach. She says, "The longer I have been in medicine, the more I understand that listening is the most important thing I do as a physician. Hospice care allows me to spend time with the patients" (p. 1031).

Spiritual care for the end of life includes activities and rituals that are appropriate to the faith tradition and support the patient through the journey from living to death. Health professionals, faith community nurses, and clergy can all be part of this spiritual care.

PALLIATIVE CARE AND HOSPICE

Palliative care is the medical subspecialty that focuses on pain relief, symptoms, and stresses of serious illness. It focuses on the quality of life rather than on the progression of an illness. Slaninka states that at any stage of a life-threatening illness, from initial symptoms to the terminal stage, the patient and family may experience a sense of loss. Loss of any sort is associated with grieving. FCNs minister to individuals and families through all stages of an illness experience. FCNs provide spiritual care, education, advocacy, and referrals for those experiencing illness, loss, and grief (Slaninka, 2006, p. 307).

Palliative care is a precursor of the principles of hospice, but it is extended to those in earlier stages of life-threatening illness and does not exclude any form of therapy. Palliative care is aimed at relieving suffering and improving quality of life for patients who are also receiving treatment for their primary condition. Such care addresses physical symptoms such as pain, shortness of breath, and nausea, but it also addresses nonphysical causes of pain, such as sadness, depression, and anxiety.

The World Health Organization definition of palliative care states that it is "an approach that improves the quality of life of patients and their families facing the problems associated with life-threatening illness, through the prevention and relief of suffering by means of early identification and impeccable assessment and treatment of pain and other problems, physical, psychosocial and spiritual."

Hospice care is holistic care provided in the home to a terminally ill person. Hospice services may begin about 6 months prior to an expected death. It is provided by a primary caregiver in the home and an interdisciplinary team consisting of a physician, nurses, a social worker, clergy, therapists (physical, music, occupational), and hospice volunteers. The FCN is an excellent addition to such a team and also can educate the congregation about both palliative care and hospice services.

The FCN's Role in Palliative and Hospice Care

Slaninka (2006) found that the more common 1 problems in palliative care include pain management and comfort, wound care, hydration and nutrition, elimination, and social isolation. The National Hospice and Palliative Care Nurses Association Position Statement (2008) states that all people have the right to optimal pain relief and that health providers have an obligation to implement appropriate pain management in a culturally sensitive manner.

The FCN does not replace the home health or hospice nurse in the home; however, the FCN can help the patient and family understand decisions that need to be made, provide referrals to appropriate resources, and give spiritual and supportive care.

Research supports the important contributions that FCNs can make in end-of-life care and show the importance of presence, prayer, religious rituals, and Scripture. FCNs can also help families grieve using the same tools. No human experience is more holistically exhausting than grieving. Families need time and support to get through the process.

═══════════*FAST FACTS in a NUTSHELL*

Resources for FCNs About Grief and Loss

Auman, M. J. (2007). Bereavement support for children. *Journal of School Nursing, 23*(1), 34–39.

Barrett, E. E. (2010). *What was lost: A Christian journey through miscarriage.* Louisville, KY: Westminster John Knox Press.

Hess, M. H. (2008). *On the road to Emmaus.* Valley Forge, PA: Judson Press.

Smith, H. I. (2007). *ABCs of healthy grieving: A companion for everyday coping* (2nd ed.). Notre Dame, IN: Ave Malcria Press.

Continued

Continued

Tedeschi, R. G., & Calhoun, L. G. (2006). Time of change? The spiritual challenges of bereavement and loss. *OMEGA, 53*(1–2): 105–116.

Weidner, H. (2006). *Grief, loss, and death: The shadow side of ministry.* Binghamton, NY: Haworth Press.

Westberg, G. E. (2004). *Good grief.* Minneapolis, MN: Augsburg Fortress.

Once a Medicare patient is admitted to hospice, all drugs, professional care, treatments, and equipment are covered. Keegan and Drick (2011) describe hospice as "possibly the best-kept secret for making an exit from physical life that is as gentle as possible" (p. 81).

Family Members

Taylor (2003) found that family caregivers expressed the need to be treated with special kindness and respect, to have communication involving both talking and listening, to be connected through active presence, to have sharing in prayer, and to have support in mobilizing faith-related resources. Stajduhar (2003) found that caregivers reported various experiences. Some reported positive benefits, stating that the caregiving experience enriched their lives, while others felt pressured to provide home care and felt exploited. The FCN can provide support across the range of these responses, supporting and encouraging those who feel enriched and finding resources for respite care or home health aides to help relieve the caregivers who feel exploited.

DEATH AT HOME

When a patient and family choose death at home, one of the most important considerations is planning and preparation. Family members must be prepared for changes that occur in the final hours of life, both to understand what is happening and to provide care. Nursing research by Kehl, Kirchohhoff, Finster, and Cleary (2008) indicates that hospice families are not routinely given complete information.

═══════════════════════*FAST FACTS in a NUTSHELL*

The most commonly distributed publications for preparing for death at home are:

- Karnes, B. (1987). *Gone from sight: The dying experience.* Depoe Bay, OR: Barbara Karns Publishing.
- Callahan, C., & Kelly, P. (1992). *Final gifts.* New York, NY: Poseidon Press.
- Houts, P. S., & Butler, J. A. (Eds.) (2003). *Caregiving: A step-by-step resource for caring for the person with cancer at home.* Atlanta, GA: American Cancer Society.

In addition to the changes that occur near death, the family must be prepared for other potential complications that will be diagnosis specific, such as massive hemorrhage. Specific instructions and plans should be in place to deal with potential complications.

Loss and Grief

Losses can be real or perceived, present or future. Many losses in palliative and hospice care settings are all too real in terms of loss of control over one's life, loss of function(s), and loss of social interaction. Significant research findings show that people with strong religious and spiritual beliefs more positively cope with end-of-life issues and dying. Dr. Harold Koenig (2002) has extensively studied the connections among religion and spirituality and health.

He contends that religious faith and the support of a faith community allow a person to have greater control over the dying process. Faith allows a person to trust that God will control circumstances based on His love, and therefore, the person can let go and "let God" (p. 20).

Deemer (2003) reports that bereavement support programs are limited by scarce resources, time, and personnel. In her survey of 450 hospices, she found the main thrust of bereavement services to be mailings of condolence letters and literature on grief.

Kissane (2004) recommends the following key components of a bereavement support program:

- Attendance at the funeral
- Expression of sympathy in cards or telephone calls
- Written information about grief
- Follow-up visits to the home
- Commemorative services during the year

The National Comprehensive Cancer Network (2004) recommends that targeted preventive support be provided to those at high risk for complicated grief. Risks include:

- A history of psychiatric illness or multiple losses
- A lack of social support
- Short hospice enrollment
- Family conflict
- Spiritual crisis
- Intensely dependent relationships

Kristjanson, Cousins, Smith, and Lewin (2005) designed and tested the four-item Bereavement Risk Index and found it reliable and valid for assessment of complicated grief. The FCN may be helpful with bereavement support and referral to appropriate community services as needed.

FAST FACTS in a NUTSHELL

Faith communities can also be affected by communal losses via accidents and natural disasters. It is a challenge to the health ministry team to coordinate memorial services and to help the faith community work through the grieving process.

15

Connecting With Community Resources

INTRODUCTION

FCNs establish connections with parishioners, colleagues, other faith communities, agencies, universities, and other organizations. Collaboration is one of the core competencies of advanced practice nursing.

In this chapter you will learn:

1. The concepts of collaboration.
2. How to build collaborations with colleagues, parishioners, other faith communities, and community-based organizations and agencies.

COLLABORATION

Collaboration is defined by Hanson and Spross (2008) as a "dynamic, interpersonal process in which two or more individuals make a commitment to each other to interact authentically and constructively to solve problems and to learn from each other in order to accomplish identified goals, purposes or outcomes. The individuals recognize and articulate the shared values that make the collaboration possible" (p. 285). This definition acknowledges that collaboration requires people to interact holistically (strengths, weaknesses, emotions) and authentically, to share power, and to remain open to the possibilities of personal and professional changes. Collaboration is a process that occurs over time. Senge, Scharmer, Jaworski, and Flowers (2004) describe collaboration as involving the head, the heart, and the will.

Faith Community Nursing: Scope and Standards of Practice (ANA–HMA, 2005) Standard 5: Implementation states that the FCN "collaborates with and empowers patients to enhance their spiritual well-being and health behaviors, reduce the occurrence of illness, modify health risk behaviors and adapt to chronic changes in health status" (p. 17). Professional Performance Standard 11: Collaboration states, "The FCN collaborates with the patient, spiritual leaders, members of the faith community, and others in the conduct of this specialized nursing practice" (p. 28). Measurement criteria for this standard include collaboration in decision making about patients' health plans; interventions, and desired outcomes; documentation of plans; and partnering with others to enhance faith-based patient care.

Underlying the concept of collaboration is the belief that quality faith community nursing care is achieved by using the gifts and talents of both the patient and health ministry team. True collaboration is a partnership without a hierarchy.

================*FAST FACTS in a NUTSHELL*

Archangelo, Fitzgerald, Carroll, and Plumb (1996), identify attributes essential for successful collaboration:

* *Trust* among all parties establishes a quality working relationship; it develops over time as the partners become acquainted.

Continued

Continued

- *Knowledge* is a necessary component for the development of trust. Knowledge and trust remove the need for supervision.
- *Shared responsibility* suggests joint decision making for patient care and outcomes as practice issues within the organization.
- *Communication* that is not hierarchal but rather two-way ensures sharing of patient information and knowledge, which improves care.
- *Cooperation and coordination* promote the use of the skills of all team members, prevent duplication, and enhance productivity.
- *Optimism* promotes success when the involved parties believe that collaboration is most effective as a means of promoting quality of care.

Barriers to collaboration can include traditions, roles, and gender stereotypes, as well as differing agendas, money issues, and differing ideas of how things should be done (Hanson & Spross, 2008). Nurses and other health care providers who are members of the faith community can also create barriers to collaboration if they do not clearly understand the FCN's role. Other health ministries may feel excluded or threatened by a new faith community nursing program. Turf issues exist in faith communities, just as they do in other settings, and hurt feelings can create barriers and cause conflict. Everyone needs to feel valued and a part of the larger mission and ministry. Good communication, as well as education, is always worth the time and energy to enhance collaborations.

CONNECTING WITH PARISHIONERS

FCNs provide counseling, expert guidance, and coaching to parishioners about a broad range of health- and illness-related issues. In doing so, FCNs serve as both educators and mentors, encouraging healthful lifestyles and behavioral changes, and thus fostering the development of others to either take the lead or share the care. Chase-Ziolek and Iris (2002) conducted a qualitative study on nurses' perspectives on the distinctive aspects of parish nursing. They report that in health counseling situations, parish nurses provide health information, deal with feelings associated with health problems, and focus on manageable goals. *Health counseling* was defined as spiritual and psychosocial support.

Olson (2000) describes the FCN's role of personal health counselor as helping people express feelings, identifying health issues that they are facing and possible solutions to them, and evaluating outcomes. Personal health counseling can occur as formal or casual encounters in any setting where the FCN and congregant meet. The personal health counselor role of the FCN is strongly supported by the literature.

Wuthnow (2004) discusses the faith community as a caring community. He states that social interaction in congregations occurs regularly over a long period of time and across a wide variety of activities. There is a distinction between "insiders" and "outsiders. Wuthnow characterizes a congregation as having a "thick" set of shared values, beliefs, understandings, traditions, and norms. As caring communities, congregations may function best by encouraging members to help each other (p. 65). The congregation as a caring community supports the ministry of faith community nursing.

CONNECTING WITH COLLEAGUES

The responsibility for care always resides with the primary provider, but consultation with another professional can confirm assessment findings and assist in planning care. Prior to consulting with others, a FCN is required by both professional standards and the Health Insurance Portability Act (HIPAA) to have the patient's permission.

======*FAST FACTS in a NUTSHELL*

Clark (2000) describes three elements of collaboration in ministry partnerships:

- *Learning:* Creative interaction between ministry professionals and congregants, which involves openness to see beyond stereotypical roles of pastor and nurse.
- *Boundaries:* Places where care and influence encounter and respect limitations, which speaks to gender roles, authority/subordination, and power and turf issues.
- *Dialogue:* Nuanced integration of insights, words, and ministry actions, a form of spiritual communication characterized by clarity of language, meekness and peacefulness, trust, and prudence (p. 132).

Hahn et al. (2001, p. 60) suggest these simple rules for effective collaboration in health ministries:

- Place God and the patient first.
- Respect one another's gifts.
- Respond to the patient's preferences and needs.
- Communicate with one another.
- Reserve territoriality for endangered species.
- Respect one another's differences.
- Communicate about mutual expectations and areas of potential overlap.
- Plan together.
- Periodically evaluate the effectiveness of working relationships.

Smith et al. (2009) describe interdisciplinary teaming, with its strong emphasis on relationship-centered care, as the "best practice" for the 21st century. They recommend that each team member ask him- or herself the following questions:

- *Are my own goals consistent with team goals?* In the faith community setting, this consistency is required to exist.

- *Do I advocate for solutions to problems that will benefit all team members?* This may or may not be relevant to faith community nursing, depending on context.
- *Do I work for consensus?* This builds the team and allows all to "own" solutions.
- *Do I cooperate with other team members' activities?* This question requires personal honesty and self-refection.
- *Do I do an equitable share of the group workload?* This question will have different answers depending upon the parish nurse model used. In a voluntary model in which the FCN provides limited hours of service, equity is not a team issue.
- *Do I support the team in dealing with larger organizational issues?* Again, consistency in goals needs to be clear in the health ministry.
- *Do I actively participate in team meetings and assignments?* Active participation in the health ministry of the faith community is an expectation of the FCN.

Smith (2003) suggests that each member of a health ministry team have a specific responsibility, and that the team meet at least monthly and be responsible for program outreach, implementation, and evaluation. The FCN brings clinical expertise and health resources to the team.

CONNECTING WITH OTHER FAITH COMMUNITIES

Connecting with other faith communities to address common health concerns or community issues provides a network of assistance for a FCN. Connections and collaborations are realistic ways of sharing human, space, and fiscal resources. Most regions of the country have interdenominational parish nurse consortia that provide strong support for FCNs and allow them to share ideas and to network.

Brudenell (2003) studied faith community nursing programs and found that collaboration between faith

communities and health organizations are successful when using a limited-domain approach to certain
defined health goals: When a goal is achieved, the collaboration ends. Gunderson (1997) also supports this
time-limited model of collaboration as a useful venue for
volunteer-driven organizations such as faith communities, as they take less time and commitment than formal
partnerships.

COLLABORATIONS WITH AGENCIES, ORGANIZATIONS, AND UNIVERITIES

Ammerman (2004) found that 83% of connections that congregations had with other organizations involving human
services were with local or regional organizations, while
17% were with national or international partners. She also
found that among congregations with any connection, there
was little difference in the proportion involved in informal
collaborations (63% had cooperative relations with religious nonprofits) or in cooperative relations with secular
nonprofits (58%). These figures were considerably higher
than the proportion of congregations involved in service
networks that included governmental units (29%), indicat-
ing that faith communities are fairly widely associated with
specialized nonprofits, and to a lesser degree, with governmental agencies. As the federal government gives more
attention to faith-based initiatives and provides them with
more resources, the proportions are likely to change in the
coming years.

Community assessment provides a FCN with a range of
resources in the community, such as health providers, universities, and other organizations. To personalize service
and make appropriate referrals, the FCN should extend his
or her network to key personnel in community agencies.
A key connection for the FCN is with the chaplain's office
and the home care department of the nearest acute care
hospital.

====================*FAST FACTS in a NUTSHELL*

Schumann and Van Duivendyk (2010) report positive effects of collaboration between hospital chaplains and FCNs:

- The link between faith and health is strengthened as congregations move toward being healing communities.
- Greater support for health ministry programs is generated as congregants share their success stories with others.
- More comprehensive care is provided as churches and hospitals work together to coordinate and provide higher levels of holistic care.
- Chaplains, FCNs, and community clergy have the opportunity to learn more about each other and their various roles with a mission of healing.

Another key connection for the FCN is the local or regional health department. Services and programs vary widely, depending upon state codes and state governmental structure. The FCN should spend at least a half day at a health department. Many departments have extensive libraries and resources for health promotion and disease prevention. The FCN must be familiar with available services and their cost to consumers. Local and state health departments post extensive epidemiological and health information on their Websites. Figure 15.1 includes examples of health department services.

Home health care services may be provided by the health department and/or nonprofit visiting nurses associations, and by proprietary home care agencies. Hospices that provide palliative care services may be free-standing or a division or department of a home health agency or acute care hospital. Responsibilities and functions of home health agencies are regulated by Medicare, private insurance companies, professional organizations, and state law.

Figure 15.1   Examples of Services Provided by
Local Health Departments

- Adult health
- Bio-terrorism response
- Birth and death records
- Child health clinics
- Dental health clinics
- Disaster management
- Environmental health
- Communicable disease control
- Family planning
- Food inspection and safety
- Health education and information
- Home safety programs
- Immunizations
- Maternal health
- Developmental disabilities
- Mental health and substance abuse
- Nursing
- School health
- Sexually transmitted disease clinics
- Tuberculosis programs

═══════════════════════════════*FAST FACTS in a NUTSHELL*

Medicare-certified agencies provide skilled professional nursing services, physical therapy, occupational therapy, social work, home health aides, and
speech pathology services. Skilled nursing care is
reimbursable by Medicare and other third parties, is
defined clearly, can only be provided by an RN, and is
goal directed. Documentation must demonstrate continued positive progress toward goals.

It is helpful for the FCN to know when congregants are discharged from skilled home health care so that he or she can address any continuing needs. Nursing students may be available to make home visits as part of community health clinical rotation.

The FCN should visit the local home health agency to review available services and costs. Special attention should be paid to programs and services that address health needs identified in the faith community assessment. For example, if a faith community has a large number of frail elderly people, services available to them should be thoroughly investigated. By developing a network of personal contacts in home health agencies, a FCN has expert consultation resources.

Nonprofit agencies and health departments have boards of directors, professional advisory committees, and ethics committees. If time permits, the FCN's service on such a board or committee puts him or her at the decision-making table and provides access to information on health-related legislation. Community participation also expands the FCNs network of resource people.

The FCN must be knowledgeable about mental health services available in the community. Such services vary widely from state to state and are almost universally inadequate to meet the needs of the community. Health insurance companies reimburse policy holders and providers considerably less for mental health services than for medical services, which has created a system where people cannot afford needed services and providers cannot afford to offer services. Many communities are without acute in-patient mental health beds as a result.

The FCN should contact the local chapter of the National Alliance for the Mentally Ill (NAMI), which has family support groups, educational programs, public campaigns to reduce stigmas, and political advocacy for mental health policy and services at all levels. The FCN should be aware of crisis intervention services, hotlines, substance abuse treatment and support groups, halfway houses, and domestic violence shelters.

The FCN must investigate and be knowledgeable about services available for senior citizens. Current demographics indicate that the size of the elderly population will explode in the next 20 years, which will affect all families and faith communities.

Other services that the FCN should be familiar with are the Department of Social Services, Social Security Administration, Department of Welfare, and food banks.

CONNECTIONS WITH ORGANIZATIONS

Health-related organizations and their Websites can provide FCNs with a wealth of information and resources. Figure 15.2 provides important Website addresses.

Figure 15.2   Health Related Resources

www.aa.org	Alcoholic Anonymous
www.alz.org	Alzheimer's Association
www.aap.org	American Academy of Pediatrics
www.aadenet.org	American Association of Diabetic Educators
www.aarp.org	American Association of Retired Persons
www.canceer.org	American Cancer Society
www.diabetes.org	American Diabetes Association
www.eatright.org	American Dietetic Association
www.americanheart.org	American Heart Association
www.lungusa.org	American Lung Association

Continued

Figure 15.2 *Continued*

www.apha.org	American Public Health Association
www.redcross.org	American Red Cross
www.arthritis.org	Arthritis Foundation
www.cdc.gov	Centers for Disease Control and Prevention
www.epa.gov	Environmental Protection Agency
www.healthfinder.gov	Health Finder
www.hospice foundation.org	Hospice Foundation of America
www.lalecheleague.org	La Leche League of America
www.lymenet.org	Lyme Disease Network
www.nami.org	National Alliance for the Mentally Ill
www.nmha.org	National Mental Health Association
www.stroke.org	National Stroke Association
www.oncolink.upenn.edu	Cancer Resources
www.planned parenthood.org	Planned Parenthood
www.hhs.gov	U.S. Dept. of Health & Human Services
www.vnaa.org	Visiting Nurse Association of America

16

Working With Vulnerable Populations

INTRODUCTION

Dr. Lu Ann Aday is a sociologist and an expert on vulnerable populations in America. She conducts research that frames issues related to health disparities and recommends policy changes to address these issues. Aday says, "To be vulnerable is to be susceptible to harm or neglect, that is, acts of commission or omission on the part of others that can wound. The word vulnerable is derived from the Latin verb vulnerare (to wound) and the noun vulnus (wound).... As members of human communities, we are all potentially vulnerable" (Aday, 2001, p. 1).

In this chapter you will learn:

1. The concept of vulnerability.
2. The demographics of vulnerable populations.
3. Resources for caring for various vulnerable populations.

THE CONCEPT OF VULNERABILITY

Vulnerability results from the combined effects of limited resources for living, which can be physical, spiritual, environmental, economic, educational, or psychological. Deficits in one area may create deficits in another area, which creates a cycle of vulnerability that may become perpetual. Vulnerable persons are at high risk for disease and adverse health events.

Poverty is the primary cause of vulnerability: It limits resources in many areas of life. Vulnerability also results from being very old or very young, or from a disease process. Vulnerability can be real or perceived. Vulnerable people have feelings of powerlessness, lack of control over their lives, depression, victimization, and disadvantage.

From a public health perspective, a population is vulnerable by virtue of status, which means that some groups are at greater risk than others (De Chesnay, 2005). FNCs may have many or few opportunities to work with vulnerable persons, depending on the demographics of the faith community.

══════════════════════════════*FAST FACTS in a NUTSHELL*

Although anyone can be vulnerable at any point in life as a result of circumstances, the following groups are vulnerable as a result of limited life resources:

- Persons living in poverty.
- Homeless persons.
- Mentally ill persons.
- Substance abusers.
- Persons dealing with domestic violence.
- Persons with disabilities.

POVERTY

Demographics

According to the U.S. Census Bureau, the poverty rate in 2009 was 14.3%, the highest rate since 1994. This translates to 43.6 million people living in poverty. The definition of *poverty* is political, and for 2009, the poverty threshold was annual earnings below $21,954 for a family of four. For children younger than 18 years of age, the poverty rate increased to 20.7% in 2009, meaning that 1 in 5 of America's children live in poverty. Approximately 25% of blacks and Hispanics are living in poverty.

Living in poverty decreases access to resources. It increases the likelihood that a person will experience adversity related to physical, psychological, and social health, as well as poor housing, nutrition, health care services, and education. More years of education and higher incomes are directly associated with better health.

Resources for FCNs

FCNs need to be knowledgeable about programs such as social services, welfare, Medicaid, Women, Infants, and Children (WIC), and the Children's Health Insurance Program (CHIP), as well as local food banks. A key role of an FCN working with people living in poverty is to connect them to resources that are available at the local level. Depending on the location, size, and resources of the faith community, reaching out to the needy may be a part of the ministry of the faith community.

HOMELESSNESS

Demographics

On any given night in America, anywhere from 700,000 to 2 million people are homeless, according to estimates of the National Law Center on Homelessness and Poverty (2004).

==*FAST FACTS in a NUTSHELL*

According to a December, 2000 report of the U.S. Conference of Mayors:

- Single men accounted for 44% of the homeless, single women 13%, families with children 36%, and unaccompanied minors 7%.
- The homeless population is about 50% African American, 35% White, 12% Hispanic, 2% Native American, and 1% Asian. (www.policyalmanac.org).

The National Coalition for the Homeless is frequently asked about the number of homeless people in the United States. They indicate that there is no easy answer to this question and that, in fact, the question itself is misleading. In most cases, homelessness is a temporary circumstance, not a permanent condition. A more appropriate measure of the magnitude of homelessness is the number of people who experience homelessness over time, not the number of "homeless people."

The National Coalition for the Homeless also indicates that most studies are limited to counting people who are in shelters or on the streets. While this approach may yield useful information about the number of people who use services such as shelters and soup kitchens, or who are easy to locate on the street, it can result in underestimates of homelessness. Many people who lack a stable, permanent residence have few shelter options because shelters are filled to capacity or are unavailable. A recent study conducted by the U.S. Conference of Mayors found that 12 of the 23 cities surveyed had to turn people in need of shelter away because of a lack of capacity. Ten of the cities experienced an increase in families with children seeking access to shelters and transitional housing, while 6 cities cited increases in the numbers of individuals seeking these resources (U.S. Conference of Mayors, 2007).

==================*FAST FACTS in a NUTSHELL*

The National Coalition for the Homeless suggests that people can help simply by "CAREing":

- Contribute.
- Advocate.
- Reach out (volunteer).
- Educate.

Resources for FCNs

Resources related to homelessness are presented in Figure 16.1.

Figure 16.1   Resources Related to Homelessness

- Annual U.S. Conference of Mayors Report on Hunger and Homelessness:
  usmayors.org
- The National Alliance to End Homelessness:
  www.endhomelessness.org
- The National Low Income Housing Coalition:
  www.nlihc.org
- The National Student Campaign Against Hunger and Homelessness:
  www.studentsagainsthunger.org/
- The National Law Center on Homelessness and Poverty:
  www.nlchp.org
- Homes for the Homeless/Institute for Children and Poverty:
  www.homesforthehomeless.com/

Continued

Figure 16.1   *Continued*

- National Health Care for the Homeless Council (formerly, The Better Homes Fund): www.nhchc.org/
- Universal Living Wage Campaign: www.universallivingwage.org
- Homeless Shelter Directory: www.homelessshelterdirectory.org
- National Housing Database for the Homeless & Low-Income: www.shelterlistings.org
- U.S. Dept. of Housing and Urban Development: hud.gov/homeless/index.cfm

17

Special Topics in Faith Community Nursing

INTRODUCTION

Mental health is integral to personal well-being. When a family is dealing with a mentally ill member, their resources can be stretched thin, both emotionally and financially. The FCN is often the only support person available to such individuals, and providing care to them can overwhelm a health ministry. To assist in serving these people and to maintain a balance of services to the rest of the congregation, the FCN needs excellent counseling skills as well as familiarity with local mental health resources and providers.

In this chapter you will learn:

1. The definition and demographics of mental illness.
2. Statistics about and FCN resources for illicit drug use and alcohol abuse.
3. Demographics and FCN resources for domestic violence and persons with disabilities.

MENTAL ILLNESS

Demographics

Mental health is defined by Healthy People 2020 as the ability to engage in productive activities and fulfilling relationships with other people, to adjust to change, and to cope with adversity. Mental health is integral to personal well-being. Healthy People 2020 defines *mental disorders* as conditions that are characterized by alterations in thinking, mood, or behavior that are associated with distress or impaired functioning.

Mental illnesses occur across the life span and affect persons of all races and all socioeconomic and educational levels. According to the National Institute of Mental Health (NIMH), about 58 million adults, or 26% of the American population, suffer from some form of mental illness. About 6%, or 1 person in 17, suffer from a mental illness that is severe and disabling. Mental illness is the leading cause of disability for people aged 15–44 and accounts for 15% of the burden of disease. One in 5 children aged 5–17 has a diagnosable mental illness. Suicide is the 10th leading cause of death, with a rate of 11.3/100,000, the highest rate being young adults aged 20–24 (12.7/100,000). Depression is a major risk factor for suicide (NIMH, 2011).

In spite of the prevalence of mental illness, Healthy People 2010 reports that only 25% of persons with mental illness receive *any* form of treatment for their illness and that a smaller percentage receives services from a mental health provider. This is clearly an outcome caused by the health insurance industry, which has historically under covered services for mental illness. Even people with "platinum" health insurance coverage find that coverage for mental disorders is limited and significantly less than coverage for physical illnesses.

===*FAST FACTS in a NUTSHELL*

Oji (2010) suggests that, among Christians, choices for psychiatric care include:

- Psychological counseling or psychotherapy alone or in conjunction with pharmacotherapy.
- Medical care with psychotherapy that incorporates faith-based counseling.
- Biblical Framework Counseling (BFC), which is based on the belief of the Bible's sufficiency to address the root cause of mental disorders and encourages counselees to continue medical care and pharmacological treatment.

Resources for FCNs

As a result of huge unmet needs, advocacy groups have become the first line of support and resources for consumers and their families. The National Alliance of the Mentally Ill (NAMI) is a consumer group that advocates for better mental health services and provides mental health education and support groups for individuals and families.

When a family is dealing with a mentally ill member, their resources can be stretched thin, both emotionally and financially, for long periods of time. The FCN is often the only support person available to such individuals, and providing care to them can overwhelm a health ministry. To assist in serving these people and to maintain a balance of services to the rest of the congregation, the FCN needs excellent counseling skills as well as familiarity with local mental health resources and providers. Resources for mental illness are provided in Figure 17.1.

Figure 17.1   Resources for Mental Illnesses

- American Association of Christian Counselors: www.aacc.net/resources
- American Association of Sociology: www.suicidology.org
- Anxiety Disorders Association of America: www.adaa.org
- Attention Deficit Information Network: addinfonetwork.com
- Bazelon Center: Legal Advocacy: www.bazelon.org
- Biblical Framework Counseling: www.biblicalframework-counseling.org
- Depression and Bipolar Support Alliance: www.ndmda.org
- Learning Disorders of America: www.ldanatl.org
- National Alliance for the Mentally Ill: www.nami.org
- National Center for Post-Traumatic Stress: www.ncptd.org
- National Center for Learning Disabilities: www.ld.org
- National Eating Disorders Association: www.openmind.org
- National Institute of Mental Health: www.nimh.nih.gov
- National Mental Health Association: www.nmha.org
- Obsessive Compulsive Foundation: www.ocf.org
- Overeaters Anonymous: www.overeatersanonymous.org
- Schizophrenics Anonymous: www.nsfoundation.org
- Spiritual Competency Resource Center: www.spiritualcompetency.com/recovery/lesson1.asp

SUBSTANCE ABUSE

Demographics

The following bulleted items are from the 2007 National Survey on Drug Use and Health (NSDUH), an annual survey sponsored by the Substance Abuse and Mental Health Services Administration (SAMHSA). The survey is the primary source of information on the use of illicit drugs, alcohol, and tobacco in the civilian, noninstitutionalized population of the United States aged 12 years or older. The survey interviews approximately 67,500 persons each year. Unless otherwise noted, all comparisons in this report described using terms such as *increased, decreased,* or *more than* are statistically significant at the 0.05 level (www.oas. samha.gov/nsduh).

Illicit Drug Use (2007)

- An estimated 19.9 million Americans aged 12 or older were current (past month) illicit drug users, meaning they had used an illicit drug during the month prior to the survey interview. This estimate represents 8% of the population aged 12 years or older. Illicit drugs include marijuana/hashish, cocaine (including crack), heroin, hallucinogens, inhalants, or prescription-type psychotherapeutics used nonmedically.
- Marijuana was the most commonly used illicit drug (14.4 million past-month users).
- There were 2.1 million cocaine users aged 12 or older, comprising 0.8% of the population. Hallucinogens were used in the past month by 1 million persons (0.4%) aged 12 or older, including 503,000 (0.2%) who had used Ecstasy.
- There were 6.9 million (2.8%) persons aged 12 or older who used prescription-type psychotherapeutic drugs nonmedically in the past month. Of these, 5.2 million used pain relievers.

- There were an estimated 529,000 users of methamphet-amine aged 12 or older (0.2% of the population).
- From 2002 to 2007, there was an increase among young adults aged 18 to 25 in the rate of use of prescription pain relievers, from 4.1% to 4.6%. There were decreases in the use of hallucinogens (from 1.9% to 1.5%), Ecstasy (from 1.1% to 0.7%), and methamphetamine (from 0.6% to 0.4%).
- Among those aged 50 to 54, the rate of past-month illicit drug use increased from 3.4% in 2002 to 5.7% in 2007. Among those aged 55 to 59, illicit drug use increased from 1.9% in 2002 to 4.1% in 2007. These trends may partially reflect the aging of the baby-boom cohort, whose lifetime rates of illicit drug use are higher than those of older cohorts.
- Among unemployed adults aged 18 or older, 18.3% were current illicit drug users.
- In 2007, there were 9.9 million persons aged 12 or older who reported driving under the influence of illicit drugs during the past year. This corresponds to 4.0% of the population aged 12 or older, similar to the rate in 2006 (4.2%), but lower than the rate in 2002 (4.7%). In 2007, the rate was highest among young adults aged 18 to 25 (12.5%).

Alcohol Use (2007)

- Slightly more than half of Americans aged 12 or older reported being current drinkers of alcohol (51.1%). This translates to an estimated 126.8 million people.
- More than one-fifth (23.3%) of persons aged 12 or older participated in binge drinking (having 5 or more drinks on the same occasion on at least 1 day in the 30 days prior to the survey). Heavy drinking was reported by 6.9% of the population aged 12 or older, or 17.0 million people.
- Past-month and binge-drinking rates among under-age persons (aged 12 to 20) have remained essentially unchanged since 2002. In 2007, about 10.7 million persons aged 12 to 20 (27.9% of this age group) reported

drinking alcohol in the past month. Approximately 7.2 million (18.6%) were binge drinkers; 2.3 million (6.0%) were heavy drinkers.

- Among persons aged 12 to 20, past-month alcohol use rates were 16.8% for Asians, 18.3% for blacks, 24.7% for Hispanics, 26.2% for those reporting two or more races, 28.3% for Native Americans, and 32.0% for whites.
- An estimated 12.7% of persons aged 12 or older drove under the influence of alcohol at least once in the past year. This percentage has decreased since 2002, when it was 14.2%. From 2006 to 2007, the rate of driving under the influence of alcohol among persons aged 18 to 25 decreased from 24.4% to 22.8%.

Resources for FCNs

Bard (2006) believes that FCNs can have a role in the prevention and management of problems associated with substance abuse. While the religious perspective of faith communities on the use of substances varies considerably, FCNs understand the culture. Connections with members of the faith community provide many opportunities for FCNs to institute programs to prevent addictions, help people to understand the problems of addiction, help provide a caring community for people suffering from addictions, and guide people to the help they need. Resources for substance abuse are presented in Figure 17.2.

Figure 17.2   Resources for Substance Abuse Treatment

- Alcoholics Anonymous: www.alcoholics-anonymous.org
- Alanon/Alateen: www.al-aanon.alateen.org

Continued

Figure 17.2   *Continued*

- American Council on Alcoholism:
  www.aca-usa.org
- Center for Substance Abuse Research:
  www.cesar.umd.edu
- Drug Abuse Resistance Education (D.A.R.E.):
  www.dare.com
- For Young Adults 17–25:
  www.strugglingyoung adults.net
- Mothers Against Drunk Driving: www.madd.org
- Narcotics Anonymous: www.na.org
- National Center for Addiction & Alcoholism:
  www.ncadd.org
- National Institute on Alcohol Abuse &
  Alcoholism: www.niaa.nih.gov
- National Institute on Drug Abuse:
  www.nida.nih.gov
- National Organization on Fetal Alcohol
  Syndrome: www.nofas.org
- National Institute on Drug Abuse for Teens:
  www.teens.drugabuse.gov

DOMESTIC VIOLENCE

Demographics

Unfortunately, domestic violence is an equal opportunity event, as it crosses all socio-economic and educational lines. *Domestic violence* is defined as physical, sexual, or psychological violence within family or intimate relationships (Brackley, 2008; Thurston et al., 2009). Abused women experience more physical and emotional impairment compared to men, and more research studies have been done on female victims. Recent research by Cook (2009) indicates that domestic violence can be mutual and that females can be dominant violence instigators. Factors found to influence whether or a not a woman stays in a relationship in which violence exists include financial resources or lack of resources, witness of parental violence, psychological factors, and police response to domestic violence (Kim & Gray, 2008).

Researchers have found that illicit drug use is much higher in persons arrested for domestic violence than among the general population and that illicit drug use is more predictive of aggression than alcohol use (Stuart et al., 2008). Depression is the most common mental health outcome of domestic violence and is diagnosed more frequently in women (Daniels, 2005).

Resources for FCNs

Routson and Hinton (2010) believe that parish nurses are in an ideal environment to support victims of domestic violence. If a parish nurse suspects that domestic violence is occurring or is approached for assistance with violence issues that are not life threatening, a parish nurse should assess the situation. If injury is involved, the parish nurse is advised to refer the person to the appropriate resource (hospital emergency department, crisis center, police). It is important to honor the confidentially of the interaction and not share any information without the express consent of the client.

═══════════════*FAST FACTS in a NUTSHELL*

Resources for domestic violence include:

- Domestic Abuse Help Line for Men and Women: www.dahmw.info/
- National Domestic Violence Hotline: www.ndvh.org

PERSONS WITH DISABILITIES

Demographics

Health, United States 2009 reports that 25% of persons 18–64 years of age had at least one basic-action difficulty (movement or emotional difficulty or vision/hearing difficulty) or complex-activity limitation (such as work or self-care limitations) in 2007, compared with 62% of adults over 65 years of age and older. An estimated 10.2 million children (13.9%) ages 0–17 years have one or more disabilities, a prevalence of 10–18.5%. This translates to 1 in 5 households having at least one child with a disability (Child and Adolescent Health Measurement Initiative [CAHMI]).

Disabilities affect major life activities, which include self-care, receptive and expressive language learning, mobility, self-direction, capacity for independent living, and financial sufficiency. The three major causes of disabilities are injuries, developmental disabilities, and chronic diseases.

Disabilities affect families in relation to the stress they cause to the family unit, the need for external resources to help the family to meet its tasks, the related financial responsibilities and responsibilities, and the social stigma (McClellan, 2004).

While churches and places of worship are exempt from the Americans with Disabilities Act, faith communities are caring communities that try to make accommodations and be inclusive of all persons. Barriers to inclusion include liability issues and lack of knowledge (Cunningham, Mulvihill, & Speck, 2009).

========================*FAST FACTS in a NUTSHELL*

Gunderson (1997) describes the following strengths of congregations:

• The strength to *accompany,* to be in the lives of others.

Continued

Continued

- The strength to *convene* interests that would not otherwise come together around a specific problems or opportunities.
- The strength to *connect* people to resources that exist in the membership.
- The power to *frame* meaning around experience and information.
- The power of *sanctuary*, providing a safe place to gather.
- The power to *bless*, to sanction.
- The power to *pray*, to find meaning between the holy and the human.
- A very *different sense of time* that gives congregations as enduring institutions the power to persist and see the community produce change.

All of the strengths listed above are strengths that FCNs can use to make the faith community a more inclusive and welcoming place for persons with disabilities. Specific resources for working with people with disabilities are presented in Figure 17.3.

Figure 17.3 Resources Related to Disabilities

- ADA Technical Assistance Program: www.adata.org
- American Association of People with Disabilities: www.aapd-dc.org
- American Council of the Blind: www.acb.org
- American Foundation for the Blind: http://www.afb.org

Continued

Figure 17.3 *Continued*

- Center for Religion and Disability:
  www.religionand disability.org
- Coalition for Citizens with Disabilities:
  www.ccd-life.org
- Lift Disability Network: www.liftdisability.net
- National Association for the Deaf: www.nad.org
- National Catholic Partnership on Disability:
  www.ncpd.org
- National Center for Birth Defects & Develop-
  mental Disabilities: www.cdc.gov/ncbddd
- National Foundation for the Blind: www.nfb.org
- National Organization on Disability: www.nod.org
- Pathways Awareness Foundation:
  www.inclusioninworship.org
- Office of Protection and Advocacy for Persons
  with Disabilities: www.ct.gov.opapd
- Persons with Disabilities Foundation:
  www.pwdf.org
- World Institute on Disability: www.wid.org
- Zachariah's Way: www.zachariahsway.com

The Scriptures of the world's religions direct people to provide for those in need. Faith communities respond to the needs of vulnerable people in many ways. Faith communities maintain food and clothing banks and participate in fundraising for organizations that provide food and shelter to the vulnerable. Whitehead et al. (2001) report that 80% of congregations offer food and cash assistance to families in their communities. FCNs use the roles of health counselor and educator to help vulnerable clients make healthful choices and learn basic life skills. An FCN can serve as an advocate and a referral agent to connect vulnerable persons to agencies that provide health and social services.

National Health Observances

Month	Target Audience
January	
National Birth Defects Prevention Month	Young adults
Glaucoma Awareness Month	Adults
National Radon Action Month	Adults
February	
American Heart Month	Adults
National Children's Dental Month	6 to 13 year olds
March	
National Colorectal Awareness Month	Adults
National Nutrition Month	Every age
April	
Alcohol Awareness Month	Teens, adults
Foot Health Awareness Month	Adults, the elderly
National Autism Awareness Month	Adults
National Youth Sports Safety Month	School-age children and teens
May	
American Stroke Month	Adults
Healthy Vision Month	Every age

Continued

Appendix   *Continued*

Month	*Target Audience*
National Asthma and Allergy Month	Children and adults
National Bike Month	Children and teens
National Arthritis Awareness Month	Adults
Skin Cancer Prevention Month	Every age
National Fitness and Sports Month	Every age
June	
Home Safety Month	Every age
July	
UV Safety Month	Every age
August	
Cataract Awareness Month	Adults, the elderly
National Immunization Awareness	Young families
September	
Fruit & Veggies: More Matters Month	Every age
National Cholesterol Education Month	Adults
Prostate Cancer Awareness Month	Adult men
October	
Halloween Safety Month	Children and parents
National Breast Cancer Awareness Month	Women
November	
American Diabetes Month	Adults
Lung Cancer Awareness Month	Adults
December	
Safe Toys and Gifts Month	Adults
National Handwashing Awareness	Children

References

Aday, L. A. (2001). *At risk in America: The health and health care needs of vulnerable populations in the United States* (2nd ed.). San Francisco, CA: Jossey Bass.

American Association of Colleges of Nursing. (2004). *AACN position statement on the practice doctorate in nursing.* Washington DC: Author.

American Nurses Association. (2001). *Code of ethics for nurses with interpretative statements.* Silver Spring, MD: Nursebooks.org.

American Nurses Association & Health Ministries Association. (2005). *Faith community nursing: Scope and standards of practice* (2nd ed.). Silver Springs, MD: Nursebooks.org.

American Nurses Association. (2010). *Nursing: Scope and standards of practice.* Silver Spring, MD: Nursebooks.org.

American Nurses Association. (2010). *Nursing's social policy statement.* Silver Spring, MD: Nursebooks.org.

Ammerman, N. T. (2004). *Pillars of faith: American congregations and their partners serving God and serving the world.* New Brunswick, NJ: Rutgers University Press.

Anderson, H. (1990). The congregation as a healing resource. In D. S. Browning, T. Job, & I. S. Evinson (Eds.), *Religious and ethical factors in psychiatric practice* (pp. 264–287). Chicago, IL: Nelson-Hall in association with the Park Ridge Center for the study of Health, Faith and Ethics.

Archangelo, V., Fitzgerald, M., Carroll, D., & Plumb, J. D. (1996). Collaborative care between nurse practitioners and primary care physicians. *Primary Care, 23*(1), 103–113.

Austin, S., Brooke, P. S., Guido, G. W., Keepnews, D. M., Michael, J. E., et al. (2004). *Nurse's legal handbook* (5th ed.). Philadelphia, PA: Lippincott, Williams & Wilkins.

Baldacchino, D., & Draper, P. (2001). Spiritual coping strategies: A review of the nursing literature. *Journal of Advanced Nursing, 34*(6), 833–841.

Bard, J. A. (2006). Faith community nurses and the prevention and management of addiction problems. *Journal of Addictions Nursing, 17*(2), 115–120.

Bastable, S. B., & Dart, M. A. (2008). Developmental stages of the learner. In S. B. Bastable (Ed.), *Nurse as educator* (3rd ed., pp.147–198). Sudbury, MA: Jones & Bartlett Publishers.

Beauchamp, T. L., & Childress, J. F. (2001). *Principles of biomedical ethics* (5th ed.). New York, NY: Oxford University Press.

Benner, P. (1999). Caring as a context for practice. In P. A. Solari-Twadell & M. A. McDermott (Eds.), *Parish nursing: Promoting whole person health within faith communities* (pp. 171–180). Thousand Oaks, CA: Sage.

Benner, P., & Wrubel, J. (1989). *The primacy of caring: Stress and coping in health and illness.* Menlo Park, CA: Addison-Wesley.

Berquist, S., & King, J. (1994). Parish nursing: A conceptual framework. *Journal of Holistic Nursing, 12*(2), 155–170.

Bishop, A. H., & Scudder, J. R. (1991). *Nursing: The practice of caring.* New York, NY: NLN Publications.

Blanchfield, C. K., & McLaughlin, E. (2006). Parish nursing: A collaborative ministry. In P. A. Solari-Twadell & M. A. McDermott (Eds.), *Parish nursing: Development, education, and administration* (pp. 65–81). St. Louis, MO: Elsevier Mosby.

Blum, H. L. (1974). *Planning for health.* New York, NY: Human Services Press.

Boss, J. G. (2004). Volunteering as a parish nurse: A response. *Parish Nurse Perspectives, 3*(1), 10.

Boyes, P. (2001). Church health fairs: Partying with a purpose. *Journal of Christian Nursing, 18*(3), 17–19.

Brackley, M. (2008). Safe family project: A training model to improve care to victims of domestic violence. *Journal of Nurses in Staff Development, 24*(1), E16–E27.

Brudenell, I. (2003). Parish nursing: Nurturing body, mind, spirit, and community. *Public Health Nursing, 20*(2), 85–94.

Bunkers, S. S. (1998). A nursing theory-guided model of health ministry: Human becoming in parish nursing. *Nursing Science Quarterly, 11*(1), 7–8.

Bunkers, S. S. (1999). Translating nursing conceptual frameworks and theory for nursing practice. In P. A. Solari-Twadell & M. A. McDermott (Eds.), *Parish nursing: Promoting whole person health within faith communities*. Thousand Oaks, CA: Sage.

Bunker, S. S., & Putnam, V. (1995). A nursing theory-based model of health ministry: Living Parse's theory of human becoming in the parish community. *Ninth Annual Westberg Parish Nurse Symposium: Parish ministering through the arts*. Northbrook, IL: Advocate Health Care.

Caiger, B. (2006). *Walking alongside: The essence of parish nursing*. Victoria, BC: Trafford Publishing.

Carroll, P. L. (2004). *Community health nursing: A practical guide*. Clifton Park, NY: Delmar.

Carson, V. B., & Koenig, H. G. (2004). *Spiritual caregiving: Healthcare as a ministry*. Philadelphia, PA. Templeton Foundation Press.

Catanzaro, A. M., Meador, K., Koenig, H. G., Kuchibhatia, M., & Clipp, E. C. (2007) Congregational health ministries: A national study of pastors' views. *Public Health Nursing, 24*(1), 6–17.

Centers for Disease Control and Prevention. Chronic disease overview. Retrieved 2010 from www.cdc.gov/chronic diseases/overview.

Centers for Disease Control and Prevention. National Center for Health Statistics. Retrieved 2011 from http://www.cdc.gov/nchs/.

Center for Health Leadership and Practice, Public Health Institute. (2011). Retrieved from www.phls.org/home/section/3–26

Chase-Ziolek, M. (2003). Rethinking our terms: Health ministry or ministry of health? *Journal of Christian Nursing, 20*(2), 21–22.

Chase-Ziolek, M. (2005). *Health, healing & wholeness: Engaging congregations in ministries of health*. Cleveland, OH: The Pilgrim Press.

Chase-Ziolek, M., & Gruca, J. (2002). Client's perceptions of distinctive aspects of nursing care received within a congregational setting. *Journal of Community Health Nursing, 17*(3), 171–183.

Chase-Ziolek, M., & Iris, M. (2002). Nurses' perspectives on the distinctive aspects of providing nursing care in a congregational setting. *Journal of Community Health Nursing, 19*(3), 173–186.

Child and Adolescent Health Measurement Initiative. (2007). Who are children with special care needs? 2005/2006. *National Survey of Children with Special Health Care Needs, Data Resource Center for Child and Adolescent Health*. Retrieved 2010 from www.childhealthdata.org.

Clark, M. B. (2000). Nurses and faith community leaders growing in partnerships. In M. B. Clark & J. K. Olson (Eds.), *Nursing within a faith community: Promoting health in times of transition.* Thousand Oaks, CA: Sage Publications.

Clark, M. B. (2000). Characteristics of a faith community. In M. B. Clark & J. K. Olson (Eds.), *Nursing within a faith community: Promoting health in ttimes of transition* (pp. 17–29). Thousand Oaks, CA: Sage.

Clark, M. B., Cary, S., Diemert, G., Ceballos, R., Sifuentes, M., Atteberry, I., Trieu, S. (2003). Involving communities in community assessment. *Public Health Nursing. 29*(6), 456–463.

Cohen, M. (1991). A comprehensive approach to effective staff development: Essential elements. Paper presented at Education Development Center, Cambridge, MA.

Corbin, J. (2000). Introduction and overview: Chronic illness and nursing. In R. Hyman and J. Corbin (Eds.), *Chronic illness: Research and theory for nursing practice* (pp. 1–15). New York, NY: Springer.

Coyle, J. (2002). Spirituality and health: Towards a framework for exploring the relationship between spirituality and health. *Journal of Advanced Nursing, 37*(6), n589–n597.

Cunningham, J. L., Mulvihill, B. A., & Speck, P. M. (2009). Disability and the church: How wide is your door? *Journal of Christian Nursing, 26*(3), 141–147.

Dahl, A. P. (2010). Faith community nursing. *Minnesota Nursing Accent,* Jan–Feb, 14–15.

Daloz, L. (1999). *Mentor: Guiding the journey of adult learners.* San Francisco, CA: Jossey Bass.

Dameron, C. (2005). Spiritual assessment made easy…with acronyms. *Journal of Christian Nursing, 22*(1), 14–15.

Daniels, K. (2005). Intimate partner violence and depression: A deadly comorbidity. *Journal of Psychosocial Nursing, 43*(1), 44–51.

Davis Lee, E. A. (2006). Zeroing in on Christian caring: Finding your model of caring practice. *Journal of Christian Nursing, 23*(3), 14–19.

Deal, B. (2008). *The lived experience of giving spiritual care.* Denton, TX: Diss: Texas Women's University.

Death with Dignity National Center. Retrieved 2010 from www.deathwithdignity.org.

De Chesnay, M. (Ed.) (2005). *Caring for the vulnerable: Perspectives in nursing theory, practice, and research.* Sudbury, MA: Jones & Bartlett.

Deemer, C. (2003). A national survey of hospice bereavement services. *OMEGA: The Journal of Death and Dying, 47*(4), 327–341.

DeNavas-Walt, C., Proctor, B. D., & Smith, J. C. (2009). U.S. Census Bureau. *Income, poverty, and human services in the U.S.* Washington, DC: U.S. Government Printing Office.

Doak, C. C., Doak, L. G., & Root, J. H. (1996). *Teaching patients with low literacy skills* (2nd ed.). Philadelphia, PA: Lippincott.

Dolan, J. A., Fitzpatrick, M. L., & Herrmann, E. K. (1983). *Nursing in society: A historical perspective* (15th ed.). Philadelphia, PA: WB Saunders Company.

Donley, R. (1991). Spiritual dimensions of health care: Nursing's mission. *Nursing & Health Care, 12*(4), 178–183.

Dueck, A. (2006). Thick patients, thin therapy and a Prozac God. *Theology News and Notes, 53*(1), 406.

Dueck, A., & Reimer, K. (2003). Retrieving the viruses in psychotherapy: Thick and thin discourse. *American Behavioral Scientist, 47*(4), 427–441.

Durban, E. (2003). Making health ministry accessible and visible: The health fair. In D. L. Patterson (Ed.), *The essential parish nurse: ABCs for congregational health ministry.* Cleveland, OH: Pilgrim Press.

Durrant, L., & Rieckmann, T. (2009). Facilitating support groups. In R. J. Bensley & J. Brookins-Fisher. *Community health education methods* (3rd ed., pp. 131–160). Sudbury, MA: Jones and Bartlett.

Dwyer, J. A. (1990). Peace. In J. A. Komonchak, M. Collins, & D. A. Lane (Eds.), *The new dictionary of theology* (pp. 748–753). Wilington, DE: Michae Gazier.

Eriksson, K. (2002). Caring science in a new way. *Nursing Science Quarterly, 15*(1), 61–65.

Ervin. N. E. (2002). *Advanced community health nursing practice: Population-focused care.* Upper Saddle River, NJ: Prentice Hall.

Evangelical Lutheran Church in America. (2010). Retrieved October 2010 from http://www.elca.org/Growing-In-Faith/Vocation/Rostered-Leadership/Diaconal-Ministry/.

Farber, A., & Farber, S. (2006). The respectful death model: Difficult conversations at the end of life. In R. S. Katz & T. A. Johnson (Eds.), *When professionals weep* (pp. 221–236). New York, NY: Routlege.

Favor, C. A. (2004). Relational spirituality and social caregiving. *Social Work, 49*(2), 241–249.

Federal Interagency Forum on Aging-Related Statistics. Older Americans 2010: Key indicators of well-being. Retrieved 2010 from www.agingstats.gov.

Fisher, E. (1999). Low literacy levels in adults: Implications for patient education. *Journal of Continuing Education in Nursing, 30*(2), 56–61.

Fitzgerald, K. (2008). Instructional methods and settings. In S. B. Bastable (Ed.), *Nurse as educator* (3rd ed., pp. 429–471). Sudbury, MA: Jones & Bartlett Publishers.

Fowler, M. (1999). Ethics as a context for practice. In P. A. Solari-Twadell & M. A. McDermott (Eds.), *Parish nursing: Promoting whole person health within faith communities* (pp. 181–194). Thousand Oaks, CA: Sage.

Fowler, M., & Peterson, B. S. (1997). Spiritual themes in clinical pastoral education. *Journal of Supervision and Training in Ministry, 18,* 46–54.

Fruh, S., & Jezek, K. (2010). Save a life, save the world. *Journal of Christian Nursing, 27*(1), 43–45.

Galek, K., Flannelly, K., Vane, A., & Galek, R. (2005). Assessing a patient's spiritual needs: A comprehensive instrument. *Holistic Nursing Practice, 19*(2), 62–69.

Garity, J., & Ryan, A. (2002). The impact of an advisory board on a parish nurse program. *Journal of Nursing Administration, 32*(12), 616–619.

George, J. B. (2006). Faith community nursing practice with clients with chronic illness. In J. S. Hickman (Ed.), *Faith community nursing* (pp. 295–306). Philadelphia, PA: Lippincott, Willliams & Wilkins .

Gilligan, C. (1982). *In a different voice.* Cambridge, MA: Harvard University Press.

Glanz, K., Rimer, B. K., & Viswanath, K. (Eds.) (2008). *Health behavior and health education* (4th ed.). San Francisco, CA: Jossey Bass.

Glaser, B., & Strauss, A. (1968). *Time for dying.* Chicago, IL: Aldine.

Gottlieb, L., & Allen, M. (1997). Developing a classification system to examine a model of nursing in primary care settings. In L. Gottlieb & H. Ezer (Eds.), *A perspective on health, family, learning, and collaborative nursing* (pp. 18–31). Montreal, QC: McGill University School of Nursing.

Green, M. L. (2001). The nurse in the community. In N. J. Brent (Ed.), *Nurses and the law* (2nd ed.). Philadelphia, PA: W. B. Saunders.

Gunderson, G. (1997). *Deeply woven roots: Improving the quality of life in your community.* Minneapolis, MN: Fortress Press.

Hansen, M., & Fisher, J. C. (1998). Patient-centered teaching from theory to practice. *American Journal of Nursing, 98*(1), 56–60.

Hanson, C. M., & Spross, J. A. (2008). The context of collaboration in contemporary health care. In A. B. Hamric & J. A. Spross (Eds.), *Advanced practice nursing: An integrative approach* (4th ed., pp. 297–314). Philadelphia, PA: Saunders.

Health Ministries Association USA. (2004). *A congregational guide to beginning and implementing a parish nursing health ministry.* http://www.pcusa.org/health/usa.

Health on the Net. (2011). Retrieved from www.healthonthenet.org

Healthy People 1990, 2000, 2010, 2020. Retrieved from www. healthy people.gov

Healthy People 2020. Retrieved from http://healthypeople.gov/2020/topicsobjectives2020/overview.aspx?topicid=28

Hickman, J. S. (2006). *Faith community nursing*. Philadelphia, PA: Lippincott Williams & Wilkins.

Hickman, J. S. (2011). An introduction to nursing theory. In J. B. George (Ed.), *Nursing theories: The base for professional practice* (6th ed.). Upper Saddle River, NJ: Pearson.

Hinton, S. T. (2010). Insights and resources toolbox. *Journal of Christian Nursing, 27*(4), 289.

HITECH Act and HIPAA. (2010). Retrieved from http://www.hipaa-survivalguide.com.

Hungelmann, J., Kenkel-Rossi, E., Klassen, L., & Stollenwerk, R. (1996). Focus on spiritual well-being: Harmonious interconnectedness of mind-body-spirit—Use of the JAREL spiritual well-being scale. *Geriatric Nursing, 17*(6), 262–266.

Hurley, J., & Mohnkern, S. (2004). Mobilize support groups to meet congregational needs. *Journal of Christian Nursing, 21*(4), 34–39.

Independent Sector. (2010). Retrieved from http://www.independent sector.org/is_announces_value_Volunteer_time_/20100412.

Institute of Medicine. (2003). *Health professions education: A bridge to quality*. Washington, DC: National Academies Press.

International Parish Nurse Resource Center. Retrieved October 2010 from www.parishnurses.org.

Johnson, R. P. (1992). *Body, mind, and spirit: Tapping the healing power within you*. Liguori, MO: Liguori Publications.

Joint Commission. (2011). Standards FAQ details. Retrieved from http.www.jointcommission.org/standards_information.jcfaq/details.aspx

Kalisch, P. A., & Kalisch, B. J. (2004). *American nursing: A history* (4th ed.). Philadelphia, PA: Lippincott Williams & Wilkins.

Keegan, L., & Drick, C. A. (2011). *End of life: Nursing solutions for death with dignity*. New York, NY: Springer Publishing.

Kehl, K. A., Kirchohhoff, K. T., Finster, M., & Cleary, J. F. (2008). Materials to prepare hospice families for dying in the home. *Journal of Palliative Medicine, 11*(7), 969–972.

Kerrigan, R., & Harkulich, J. T. (1993). A spiritual tool. *Health Progress, 74*(5), 46–49.

Kissane, D. (2004). Bereavement support services. In S. Payne, J. Seymour, & C. Ingleton (Eds.), *Palliative care nursing: Principles and evidence for practice* (pp. 539–554). Berkshire, England: Open University Press.

Knowles, M. S., Holton, E. F., & Swanson, R. A. (1998). *The adult learner: The definitive classic in adult education and human response development* (5th ed.). Houston, TX: Gulf Publishing.

Koenig, H. G. (2002). A commentary: The role of religion and spirituality at the end of life. *The Gerontologist, 42*, 20.

Koenig, H. G. (2002). An 83-year-old woman with chronic illness and strong religious beliefs. *Journal of the American Medical Association, 288*(4), 487–493.

Koenig, H. G. (2007). *Spirituality in patient care: Why, how, when, and what.* Philadelphia, PA: Templeton Foundation Press.

Koenig, H. G., McCullough, M. E., & Larson, D. B. (2001). *Handbook of religion and health.* New York, NY: Oxford University Press.

Kreps, G. L., Barnes, M. D., & Thackeray, R. (2009). Health communication. In R. J. Bensley & J. Brookins-Fisher (Eds.), *Community health education methods* (3rd ed., pp. 73–102). Sudbury, MA: Jones & Bartlett.

Kreutzer, S. (2010). Nursing body and soul in the parish Lutheran deaconess motherhouses in Germany and the United States. *Nursing History Review, 18*, 134–150.

Kristjanson, L. J., Cousins, K., Smith, J., & Lewin G. (2005). Evaluation of the Bereavement Risk Index (BRI): A community hospice care protocol. *International Journal of Palliative Nursing, 11*(12), 610–618.

Lachman, V. D. (2009). Practical use of the nursing code of ethics. *MEDSURG Nursing, 18*(1), 55–57.

Lampe, S. S. (1985). Focus charting: Streamlining documentation. *Nursing Management, 16*(7), 43–44.

Lankarani-Fard, A., Knapp, H., Lorenz, K. A., Golden, J. F., Taylor, A., Feld, J. E., Asch, S. M. (2010). Feasibility of discussing end-of-life care goals with inpatients using a structured, conversational approach: The go wish card game. *Journal of Pain Symptom Management, 39*(4), 637–643.

LaRocca-Pitts, M. (2008). FACT: Taking a spiritual history in a clinical setting. *Journal of Health Care Chaplaincy, 15*(1), 1–12.

Leininger, M. (Ed.) (1984). *Care: The essence of nursing and health.* Thorofare, NJ: Slack.

Lindberg, C. (1986). The Lutheran tradition. In R. L. Members & D. W. Amundsen (Eds.), *Caring and curing: Health and medicine in Western religious traditions* (pp. 5–39). New York, NY: Macmillan.

Locker, D. (2010). *The volunteer book: A guide for churches and non-profits.* Kansas City, MO: Beacon Hill.

Lorig, K., Holman, H., Sobel, D., Gonzalez, V., & Minor, M. (2006). *Living a healthy life style with chronic conditions.* Boulder, CO: Bull Publishing Company.

Lubkin, I. M., & Larsen, P. D. (2005). *Chronic illness: Impact and interventions* (6th ed.). Sudbury, MA: Jones & Bartlett.

Maddox, M. (2001). Circle of Christian caring: A model for parish nursing practice. *Journal of Christian Nursing, 18*(3), 11–13.

Matthews, D. A., McCullough, M. E., Larson, D. B., Koenig, H. G., Swyers, J. P., & Milano, M. G. (1998). Religious commitment and health status. *Archives of Family Medicine, 7*, 118–124.

Mayhugh, L. J., & Martens, K. H. (2001). What's a parish nurse to do? Congregational expectations. *Journal of Christian Nursing, 18*(3), 14–16.

McDermott, M. A. (1999). Accountability and rationale. In P. A. Solari-Twadell & M. A. McDermott (Eds.), *Parish nursing: Promoting whole health within faith communities* (pp. 227–232.). Thousand Oaks, CA: Sage.

McKnight, J. L., & Kretzmann, J. P. (1997). Mapping community capacity. In M. Minkler (Ed.), *Community organizing and community building for health* (pp. 157–172). New Brunswick, NJ: Rutgers University Press.

McLaughlin, G. H. (1969). SMOG-grading: A new reading ability formula. *Journal of Reading, 12*(8), 639–646.

Metzger, S. (2006). Working in a faith community. In J. S. Hickman (Ed.), *Faith community nursing* (pp. 75–91). Philadelphia, PA: Lippincott, Williams & Wilkins.

Meyer, P. A. (1996). Management fundamentals for parish nurse program directors. *Perspectives in Parish Nurse Practice, 1*, 3–6.

Miller, L. W. (1997). Nursing through a lens of faith: A conceptual model. *Journal of Christian Nursing, 14*(1), 17–21.

Milton, C. L. (2008). Accountability in nursing: Reflecting on ethical codes and professional standards of nursing practice from a global perspective. *Nursing Science Quarterly, 21*(4), 300–303.

Morrison, G. W. (2001). *Early childhood education today* (8th ed.). Upper Saddle River, NJ: Merrill Prentice Hall.

National Coalition for the Homeless. Retrieved 2010 from www.nationalhomeless.org.

National Comprehensive Cancer Network. (2004). *NCCN Clinical Practice Guidelines in Oncology: Palliative Care.* Retrieved 2010 from www.nccn.org/professionals/physician_gls/PDF/palliative.pdf.

National Hospice and Palliative Care Nurses Association Position Statement. (2008). Retrieved 2011 from http://www.nhpco.org/templates/1/homepage.cfm

National Institute of Mental Health. (2011). Retrieved from www.nimh.gov

The National Law Center on Homelessness and Poverty. (2004). *Homelessness in the United States and the human right to housing.* Washington, DC: Author.

Nease, B. (2010). Master mentor and connoisseur coach: Learn from the best. *Journal of Christian Nursing, 27*(4), 2322–2324.

O'Brien, M. E. (2003). *Parish nursing: Healthcare ministry within the church.* Sudbury, MA: Jones & Bartlett Publishers.

O'Brien, M. E. (2008). *Spirituality in nursing: Standing on holy ground.* Boston, MA: Jones & Bartlett Publishers.

O'Brien, M. E. (2011). *Spirituality in nursing: Standing on holy ground.* Sudbury, MA: Jones & Bartlett.

Oji, V. (2010). Mind, medications, and mental disorders: A spiritual approach. *Journal of Christian Nursing, 27*(2), 76–83.

Olson, J. K. (2000). Functions of the nurse as health promoter in a faith community. In M. B. Clark & J. K. Olson (Eds.), *Nursing in a faith community: Promoting health in times of transition.* Thousand Oaks, CA: Sage.

Otterness, N., Gehrke, P., & Sener, I. M. (2007). Partnerships between nursing education and faith communities: Benefits and challenges. *Journal of Nursing Education, 46*(1), 39–44.

Pierce, L. L., & Lutz, B. J. (2005). In I. M. Lubkin & P. D. Hansen (Eds.), *Chronic illness: Impact and interventions* (6th ed., pp. 220–230). Sudbury, MA: Jones & Bartlett.

Parker, M. (2000). Mobilizing volunteers for service. *Healing Hearts and Hands, 4*(3), 1.

Parker, W. (2004). How well do parish nurses document? *Journal of Christian Nursing, 21*(2), 13–14.

Parse. R. R. (1998). *The human becoming school of thought.* Thousand Oaks, CA: Sage.

Parse, R. R. (2007). A humanbecoming perspective on quality of life. *Nursing Science Quarterly, 20,* 308–311.

Patterson, D. L. (2003). *The essential parish nurse: ABCs for congregational health ministry.* Cleveland, OH: Pilgrim Press.

Patterson, D. L. (2007). Eight advocacy roles for parish nurses. *Journal of Christian Nursing, 24*(1), 33–35.

Pender, N. J., Murdaugh, C. L., & Parsons, M. A. (2011). *Health promotion in nursing practice* (6th ed.). Upper Saddle River, NJ: Prentice Hall.

Polit, D. E., & Beck, C. T. (2008). *Nursing research: Generating and assessing evidence for nursing practice* (8th ed.). Philadelphia, PA: Lippincott Williams & Wilkins.

Puchalski, C. M., & Romer, A. L. (2000). Taking a spiritual history allows clinicians to understand patients more fully. *Journal of Palliative Medicine, 3*, 129–137.

Rao, J. K., Anderson, L. A., & Smith, S. M. (2002). End of life is a public health issue. *American Journal of Preventive Medicine, 23*(3), 215–220.

Ratzan, S. C., & Parker, R. M. (2000). Introduction. In C. R. Selden, M. Zorn, S. C. Ratzan, & R. M. Parker (Eds.), *National Library of Medicine current bibliographies in medicine: Health literacy.* Bethesda, MD: NIH, USDHHS.

Reed, P. G. (1991). Preferences for spiritually related nursing interventions among terminally ill and non-terminally ill hospitalized adults and well adults. *Applied Nursing Research, 4*(3), 122–137.

Reinhard, S. C., Grossman, J., & Piren, K. (2004). Advocacy and the advanced practice nurse. In L. A. Joel (Ed.), *Advanced nursing practice: Essentials for role development.* Philadelphia, PA: FA Davis.

Routson, J. L., & Hinton, S. T. (2010). Domestic violence and the role of the parish nurse. *Journal of Christian Nursing, 27*(4), 302–305.

Rydholm, L. (2006). Documenting the value of faith community nursing. *Creative Nursing, 2*, 10–12.

Sage, B. (2008). Health ministries network. *Health Ministries News, 13*(1), 15.

Schoonover-Shoffner, K. (2002). Does "adjusting" go far enough? *Journal of Christian Nursing, 19*(3), 12–13.

Schroll, A. (2010). Choosing hospice. *Journal of Palliative Medicine, 13*(8), 1031.

Schumann, R., & VanDuivendyk, T. (2010). Connections, collisions, and complementarity: The dynamic of health care chaplain, parish nurse and parish clergy collaboration. *Journal of Health Care Chaplaincy, 11*(2), 61–67.

Senge, P. M., Scharmer, C.O., Jaworski, J., & Flowers, B. S. (2004). *Presence: An exploration of profound change in people, organizations, and society.* New York, NY: Currency/Doubleday.

Sessanna, L., Finnell, D., & Jezewski, M. A. (2007). Spirituality in nursing and health related literature: A concept analysis. *Journal of Holistic Nursing, 25*(4), 252–262.

Shelly, J. A., & Fish S. (1988). *Spiritual care: The nurse's role* (3rd ed.). Downers Grove, IL: InterVarsity Press.

Shelly, J. A., & Miller, A. B. (1999). *Called to care: A Christian theology of nursing.* Downers Grove, IL: InterVarsity Press.

Shuster, G. F., & Goeppinger, J. (2008). Community as client: Assessment and analysis. In M. Stanhope & J. Lancaster (Eds.), *Public health nursing: Population-centered healthcare in the community* (7th ed., pp. 340–372). St. Louis, MO: Mosby.

Slaninka, S. C. (2006). Faith community nursing practice and palliative care, grief, and loss. In J. S. Hickman (Ed.), *Faith community nursing* (pp. 307–321). Philadelphia, PA: Lippincott, Williams, & Wilkins.

Slutz, M. (2010). Liability issues for parish nurses and faith communities. *Parish Nurse Perspectives, 9*(1), 9–10.

Smith, S. D. (2000). Parish nursing: A call to integrity. *Journal of Christian Nursing, 17*(1), 18–21.

Smith, S. D. (2003). *Parish nursing: A handbook for the new millennium.* New York, NY: Haworth Pastoral Press.

Smith, T. D., Vezina, M. L., & Samost, M. E. (2000). Mediated roles: Working with other people. In L. A. Joel (Ed.), *Advanced practice nursing: Essentials for role development* (2nd ed.). Philadelphia. PA: F.A. Davis.

Solari-Twadell, P. A., & Hackbarth, D. P. (2010). Evidence for a new paradigm of the ministry of parish nursing practice using the nursing intervention classification. *Nursing Outlook, 58*(2), 69–75.

Spache, G. (1953). A readability formula for primary grade reading materials. *Elementary School Journal, 53*(7), 410–413.

Stajduhar, K. I. (2003). Examining perspectives of family members involved in the delivery of palliative care at home. *Journal of Palliative Care, 19*(1), 27–35.

Stanford University School of Medicine. Chronic Disease Self-Management Program. Retrieved 2010 from http://patienteduction.stanford.edu.

Stegmeir, D. (2002). Faith & nursing: Adjusting nursing theories to Christian beliefs. *Journal of Christian Nursing, 19*(3), 11–15.

Sternberg, E. M. (2009). *Healing spaces: The science of place and well-being.* Cambridge, MA: Harvard University Press.

Stoll, R. I. (1989). Spirituality and chronic disease. In V. B. Carson (Ed.), *Spiritual dimensions of nursing practice* (pp. 180–216). Philadelphia, PA: W.B. Saunders.

Stuart, G., Temple, J., Follansbee, W., Bucossi, M., Hellmuth, J., & Moore, T. (2008). The role of drug use in a conceptual model of intimate partner violence in men and women arrested for domestic violence. *Psychological Addict Behavior, 22*(1), 12–24.

Stuckey, J. C. (2001). Blessed assurance: The role of religion and spirituality on Alzheimer's disease caregiving and other significant life events. *Journal of Aging Studies, 15*(1), 69–84.

Swinney, J., Anson-Wonkka, C., Maki, E., & Corneau, J. (2001). Community assessment: A church community and the parish nurse. *Public Health Nursing, 18*(1), 40–66.

Tang, T. S., Funnell, M. M., & Anderson, R. M. (2006). Group education strategies for diabetes self-management. *Diabetes Spectrum, 19*(2), 99–105.

Taylor, E. J. (2003). Nurses caring for the spirit: Patients with cancer and family caregiver expectations. *Oncology Nursing, 30*(4), 585–590.

Thurston, W., Tutty, L., Eisener, A., Lalonde, L., Belenky, C., & Osbourne, B. (2009). Implementation of universal screening for domestic violence in a urgent care community health center. *Health Promotion Practice, 10*(4), 517–526.

Tillett, J. (2005). Adolescents and informed consent: Ethical and legal issues. *Journal of Perinatal & Neonatal Nursing, 19*(2), 112–121.

Todd, J., & Baldwin, C. (2006). An opinion on death and dying: A picture worth painting. *Journal of Multicultural Nursing, 12*(2), 54–55.

Tong, R. (2011). Feminist ethics: Some applicable thoughts for advanced practice nurses. In J. B. Butts & K. L. Rich (Eds.), *Philosophies and theories for advanced nursing practice* (pp.165–184). Sudbury, MA: Jones & Bartlett Learning.

Tuck, I., Wallace, D., & Pullen, L. (2001). Spirituality and spiritual care provided by parish nurses. *Western Journal of Nursing Research, 23*(5), 441–453.

U.S. Commission on Consumer Protection and Quality in the Health Care Industry (1998). Consumer Bill of Rights and Responsibilities. www.hcquality.gov/final/apenda.html.

U.S. Conference of Mayors. (2007). A Hunger and Homelessness Survey. Retrieved 2010 from www.usmayors.org.

Ustal, D. B. (2003). The ethic of care: A Christian perspective. *Journal of Christian Nursing, 20*(4), 13–17.

Van Dover, L., & Pfeiffer, J. B. (2006). Spiritual care in Christian parish nursing. *Journal of Advanced Nursing, 57*(2), 213–221.

Van Loon, A., & Carey, L. B. (2002). Faith community nursing and health care chaplaincy in Australia: A new collaboration. In L. Vandecreek & S. Mooney (Eds.), *Parish nurses, health care chaplains and community clergy: Navigating the maze of professional relationships.* New York, NY: Haworth Press.

Wallace, D. C., Tuck, I., Boland C. S., & Witucki, J. M. (2002). Client perceptions of parish nursing. *Public Health Nursing, 19*(2), 128–135.

Wasserman, L. S. (2008). Respectful death: A model for end-of-life care. *Clinical Journal of Oncology Nursing, 12*(4), 621–626.

Watson, J. (1985). *Nursing: Human science and human care.* Norwalk, CT: Appleton Century Crofts.

Weis, D. M., Schank, M. J., Coenan, A., & Matheus, R. (2002). Parish nursing practice with client aggregates. *Journal of Community Health Nursing, 19*(2), 105–113.

Westberg, G. (1982). The church as a health place. *Dialog, 27*(3), 189–191.

Westberg, G. (1999). A personal historical perspective of whole person health and the congregation. In P. A. Solari-Twadell & M. A. McDermott (Eds.), *Parish nursing: Promoting whole person health and the congregation.* Thousand Oaks, CA: Sage.

Westburg, G. E., & Westburg McNamara, J. (1990). *The Parish Nurse: Providing a minister of health for your congregation.* Minneapolis, MN: Augsburg Press.

World Health Organization. (1948). *Preamble to the Constitution of the World Health Organization.* Author.

World Health Organization. (2011). Retrieved from www.who.org

Wilson, R. P. (1997). What does the parish nurse do? *Journal of Christian Nursing, 14*(1), 13–16.

Wilson, L. (2000). Implementation and evaluation of church-based health fairs. *Journal of Community Health Nursing, 17*(1), 39.

Wurzbach, M. E. (Ed.) (2004). *Community health education and promotion* (2nd ed.). Sudbury, MA: Jones & Bartlett.

Wuthnow, R. (2004). *Saving America: Faith-based services and the future of civil society.* Princeton, NJ: Princeton University Press.

Ziebarth, D. J. (2006). Innovation fosters community health. *Creative Nursing, 12*(2), 6–7.

Ziebarth, D. J. (2007). Specialty practice celebrates 10 years of caring. *Nursing Matters, 18*(1), 21.

Ziebarth, D. (2006). Policies and procedures for the ministry of parish nursing practice. In P. A. Solari-Twadell & M. A. McDermott (Eds.), *Parish nursing: Development, education, and administration* (pp. 257–267). St. Louis, MO: Elsevier Mosby.

Ziebarth, D. J., & Miller, C. L. (2010). Exploring parish nurses' perspectives of parish nurse training. *Journal of Continuing Education in Nursing, 41*(6), 273–280.

Index

Printed in the United States
By Bookmasters